HEALTH
RESEARCH

Essential Link to Equity in Development

COMMISSION MEMBERS

John R. Evans (Canada), Chair
Gelia T. Castillo (the Philippines), Deputy Chair
Fazle Hasan Abed (Bangladesh)
Sune D. Bergstrom (Sweden)
Doris Howes Calloway (United States)
Essmat S. Ezzat (Egypt)
Demissie Habte (Ethiopia)
Walter J. Kamba (Zimbabwe)
Adetokunbo O. Lucas (Nigeria)
Adolfo Martinez-Palomo (Mexico)
Saburo Okita (Japan)
V. Ramalingaswami (India)

HEALTH RESEARCH

Essential Link to Equity in Development

The Commission on Health Research for Development

Oxford University Press

Oxford University Press

Oxford New York Toronto
Delhi Bombay Calcutta Madras Karachi
Petaling Jaya Singapore Hong Kong Tokyo
Nairobi Dar es Salaam Cape Town
Melbourne Auckland

and associated companies in
Berlin Ibadan

Copyright © 1990
by the Commission on Health Research for Development
22 Plympton Street, Cambridge, MA 02138, U.S.A.
Published for the Commission on Health Research for Development by
Oxford University Press, 200 Madison Avenue, New York, NY 10016

Oxford is a registered trademark of Oxford University Press.

Library of Congress Cataloging-in-Publication Data:
Commission on Health Research for Development.
Health research.
Includes bibliographical references.
1. Public health—Research—Developing countries.
2. Medical care—Research—Developing countries.
I. Title.
RA441.5.C63 1990 362.1'07201724 90-6872
ISBN 0-19-520838-2

Printing (last digit): 9 8 7 6 5 4 3 2 1
Printed in the United States of America
on acid-free paper

FOREWORD

The Commission on Health Research for Development, an independent international initiative, was formed in late 1987 with the aim of improving the health of people in developing countries. We focused on research in the belief that it has enormous—and, in great part, neglected—power to accomplish that goal.

Research uses the scientific method to discover facts and their interrelationships and then to apply this new knowledge in practical settings. This process was the means by which the jet engine was invented, the atom split, and the green revolution of the past 25 years generated. Research holds the same promise for health, a promise that we have seen fulfilled with the development of new tools such as antibiotics for the treatment of disease, vaccines for its prevention, and insecticides for controlling the vectors that transmit it. Yet for the world's most vulnerable people, the benefits of research offer a potential for change that has gone largely untapped. The Commission's mandate was to survey current research on the health problems of developing countries, identify strengths and weaknesses, and propose improvements wherever we saw the greatest opportunities.

This book, the result of our work, represents the ideas and experience of many people. Over 24 months, we reviewed available information, commissioned special papers, and consulted widely around the world. At eight Commission meetings, held in the Federal Republic of Germany, Zimbabwe, the United States, Mexico, India, Japan, France, and Sweden, we invited local and international experts in health and development to share their experiences and observations with us. We heard from health researchers, social activists, and administrators, and met with ministers of health and representatives of WHO and UNICEF. We convened regional workshops in Bangladesh, Zimbabwe, Brazil, Egypt, and Mexico in order to hear diverse viewpoints and to shape a broad-based agenda for change. And both commissioners and staff met individually with hundreds of health and development experts around the world.

We commissioned case studies of health research activities, research capacity, and support for research in 10 developing countries— Bangladesh, Brazil, Egypt, Ethiopia, India, Mali, Mexico, the Philippines, Thailand, and Zimbabwe. We commissioned papers and held workshops focused on subjects of particular interest. These were attended by a wide range of researchers and program directors. Our small staff produced a number of background papers and undertook a survey, the first of its kind, of global research on the health problems of developing countries and a study of the main resource flows supporting it. This has produced an extraordinary range of useful information on how research on the health problems of developing countries is financed, where it is done, and how it is promoted.

The Commission itself has a global point of view. Eight of our 12 members come from developing countries: Bangladesh, Ethiopia, Egypt, India, Mexico, Nigeria, the Philippines, and Zimbabwe. Four come from industrialized countries: Canada, Japan, Sweden, and the United States. Most of us have been actively involved with biomedical, social, or epidemiological research, and several have had important responsibilities for institutional development in government, universities, medical schools, and research institutions. Besides health experts, we have a businessman, a nutritionist, an economist, a rural sociologist, and a lawyer to broaden our perspective.

The Commission is independent, not the creature of any agency or institution. Since it was not created by a government or an international agency, it is free to reflect frankly on the policies and practices of all. The Commission was created, in fact, by its sponsors, a diverse group of 16 donors from Europe, North America, Asia, and Latin America. Special acknowledgment is due the Edna McConnell Clark Foundation (United States), the International Development Research Centre (Canada), and the Gesellschaft für Technische Zusammenarbeit (Federal Republic of Germany), which provided the leadership in launching the Commission. Although no single funder has supplied more than 12 percent of the Commission's budget, representatives from these three agencies played invaluable roles in launching and nurturing our work.

In our exchanges, one fundamental relationship we explored was the relationship between health and development. The multidisciplinary character of the Commission's membership helped to shape a shared vision that good health can be a driving force for national development.

From the start, all of us concurred that research is an essential but often neglected link between aspiration and action. Our most difficult internal dialogue, not unexpectedly, revolved around the many ways that research can be defined and applied to furthering human health. We agreed that research to support informed and intelligent decision-making for health action deserves the highest priority. We also recognized the enormous importance of strengthening all scientists, particularly those in developing countries, to participate in the effort to advance the frontiers of basic knowledge. Our debate was not whether these were incompatible objectives but how priorities should and could be set.

This report, based on our analysis and deliberations, represents a consensus on what must be done to realize the potential of research for furthering world health. The book has three main sections. In Part One we review the profound global inequities in health and argue that health is not only a beneficiary of development but a spur to it as well. Then we discuss why research is needed in the effort to improve Third World health. Part Two sets out the findings of our survey and country studies, examining how health research on developing-country health problems is financed, which health problems are studied, where it is done, and how it is promoted. Part Three draws conclusions and summarizes our recommendations for action.

We believe, in the end, that health for all people depends on many things: on commitment to the goal; on the political will to push for it; on programs to reach all the people, particularly the most vulnerable; on resources to support those programs—and on knowledge. This book presents the case for what that last element, knowledge, can do to improve the health of people who live in developing countries.

The analysis and vision represented in these pages rest on the work of many people, but the judgments are the responsibility of the 12 of us who form the Commission and the superb secretariat, led by Lincoln Chen and David Bell, with whom we worked. Respectfully we submit our report to the people it most concerns: to scientists and leaders in the Third World, who are engaged in heroic efforts to improve the health and better the life of their people; to scientists and leaders in the industrialized countries, who in an ever-shrinking world are tied to the people of developing countries by self-interest as well as humanitarian concern; and above all to the citizens of developing countries around the world, who seek a better life.

FOR THE COMMISSION
JOHN EVANS, CHAIR

CONTENTS

Boxes, Figures, and Tables

Boxes

FIGURES

TABLES

ACRONYMS AND ABBREVIATIONS

Organizations and Programs

ACC/SCN	UN Administrative Committee on Coordination—Subcommittee on Nutrition
ACHR	Advisory Committee on Health Research (WHO)
BOSTID	Board on Science and Technology for International Development
BRAC	Bangladesh Rural Advancement Committee
CARE	Cooperative for American Relief Everywhere
CAREC	Caribbean Epidemiology Center
CDC	Centers for Disease Control (U.S. Public Health Service)
CDD	Programme for Control of Diarrhoeal Diseases
CEPIS	Pan American Center for Sanitary Engineering and Environmental Sciences
CFNI	Caribbean Food and Nutrition Institute
CGIAR	Consultative Group on International Agricultural Research
CIMMYT	International Maize and Wheat Center
EC	European Community
EPI	Expanded Programme on Immunization (WHO)
FAO	Food and Agriculture Organization
FHI	Family Health International
FIELDLINCS	Field Linkages for Intervention and Control Studies (TDR)
GPA	Global Program on AIDS (WHO)
GTZ	Deutsche Gesellschaft für Technische Zusammernarbeit
HIID	Harvard Institute for International Development
HRP	Special Programme for Research, Development, and Research Training in Human Reproduction (UNDP/World Bank/WHO)
HSR	Health Systems Research (WHO)
IARC	International Agency for Research on Cancer
IBPGR	International Board for Plant Genetic Resources
ICDC	International Child Development Centre
ICDDR,B	International Centre for Diarrhoeal Disease Research (Bangladesh)
IDRC	International Development Research Centre of Canada
IFPRI	International Food Policy Research Institute
IHPP	International Health Policy Program
IMF	International Monetary Fund
INCAP	Institute of Nutrition of Central America and Panama
INCLEN	International Clinical Epidemiology Network
INRUD	International Network for the Rational Use of Drugs
IOM	Institute of Medicine (U.S. National Academy of Sciences)
IPPF	International Planned Parenthood Federation
IRRI	International Rice Research Institute
ISNAR	International Service for National Agricultural Research
IUATLD	International Union Against Tuberculosis and Lung Disease
IUNS	International Union of Nutritional Scientists
JICA	Japan International Cooperation Agency
MEAwards	Middle East Awards Program in Population and Development

MEM	Mass Education Movement (China)
NEBT	National Epidemiology Board of Thailand
NIAID	National Institute of Allergy and Infectious Disease (NIH)
NIH	U.S. National Institutes of Health
OCCGE	Organisation de Coordination et de Coopération pour la Lutte contre les Grandes Endémies
OCEAC	Organisation de Coordination et de Coopération pour la Lutte contre les Grandes Endémies en Afrique Centrale
OCP	Onchocerciasis Control Programme
OECD	Organization for Economic Cooperation and Development
ORPD	Office for Research Promotion and Development (WHO)
OTEP	Oral Therapy Extension Program (BRAC)
PAHO	Pan American Health Organization
PATH	Program for Appropriate Technology in Health
PIDS	Philippine Institute of Development Studies
RAWOO	Advisory Council for Scientific Research in Development Problems (The Netherlands)
SAARC	South Asian Association for Regional Cooperation
SADCC	Southern African Development Coordination Conference
SAREC	Swedish Agency for Research Cooperation with Developing Countries
SEAMEO	Southeastern Asian Ministers of Education Organization
SNI	National Researchers System (Mexico)
TAC	Technical Advisory Committee (CGIAR)
TDR	Special Programme for Research and Training in Tropical Diseases (UNDP/World Bank/WHO)
TROPMED	Tropical Medicine and Public Health Project (SEAMEO)
UNDP	United Nations Development Programme
UNESCO	United Nations Educational, Scientific and Cultural Organization
UNFPA	United Nations Fund for Population Activities
UNICEF	United Nations Children's Fund
UNU	United Nations University
USAID	United States Agency for International Development
WHO	World Health Organization

Abbreviations and Technical Terms

AIDS	Acquired Immune Deficiency Syndrome
DDT	Dichloro-diphenyl-trichloroethane
GDP	Gross domestic product
GNP	Gross national product
ENHR	Essential national health research
HIV	Human Immunodeficiency Virus
HFA	Health for All
NGO	Nongovernmental organization
ODA	Official development assistance
PHC	Primary health care
R&D	Research and development
STD	Sexually transmitted disease
TB	Tuberculosis
$	U.S. dollars

Executive Summary

HEALTH RESEARCH: ESSENTIAL LINK TO EQUITY IN DEVELOPMENT

Our world has become a global health village, generating an urgent need for mutual learning and joint action. The world has entered this era of health interdependence, paradoxically, at a time when the economic gap between rich and poor is widening and there are tragic inequalities in health worldwide. Life itself, our most precious gift, is almost one-third shorter in the developing world than in industrialized countries. Both health and development are undermined by high death rates of children: this hinders the transition from high to low fertility which is essential for slowing rates of population growth. Overcoming the disparities in health status is critical not only to reduce physical and emotional suffering, but also to advance individual, family, community, and national development.

As the 1990s begin, the objective of advancing health in the developing world faces formidable obstacles. One powerful tool to overcome these hindrances, a tool that is under-recognized and neglected, is research. Research is an essential key to enable people in diverse circumstances to apply solutions that are already available, and to generate new knowledge to tackle problems for which solutions are not yet known. Research is essential both to facilitate health action and to generate new understanding and fresh interventions.

One view considers that research must wait until current health service priorities have been met and financial resources are less constrained. We on this Commission consider that, on the contrary, research is essential today because the results are needed now to empower those who must accomplish more with fewer resources.

We have found a gross mismatch between the burden of illness, which is overwhelmingly in the Third World, and investment in health research, which is overwhelmingly focused on the health problems of the industrialized countries. Developing countries need stronger scientific and institutional capacity to address problems unique to their circumstances, but sufficient investment is not being made to build and sustain their health research capacity. Especially weak are the critical fields of epidemiology, the policy and social sciences, and management research. Biomedical and clinical research are somewhat stronger, but capacity-strengthening efforts in these fields are modest in scale and narrowly targeted.

International support for research on Third World problems is focused primarily on human reproduction and contraception, tropical diseases, diarrhea, and AIDS. Comparatively neglected are acute respiratory infections, tuberculosis, sexually transmitted diseases other than AIDS, injuries, chronic degenerative diseases, and mental and behavioral problems, all of which are major causes of death and disability. New and rising threats such as substance abuse and occupational and environmental hazards barely appear on the research agenda. Research is also badly neglected on problems not classified as diseases, such as health information systems, costs and financing, and the wasteful misuse of drugs. Especially lacking is support for research that informs health policy, management, and resource allocation decisions, research that we believe is essential in every country.

We propose a set of strategies through which the power of research can be harnessed to accelerate health improvements and to overcome health disparities worldwide. Health must be accorded a higher priority in national development plans. Research must be recognized as a powerful tool for health and development. The capacity of researchers and institutions must be strengthened to address local problems more effectively. Scientists around the world must be enabled to work together in stronger collaboration to attack health problems jointly. These strategies can accelerate health progress even in the face of current financial constraints and can help overcome the gross inequity in health status between the privileged and the poor.

We envisage a pluralistic, worldwide health research system that will nurture productive national scientific groups linked together in transnational networks to address both national and global health problems. We offer four major recommendations toward realizing that vision:

1. All countries should vigorously undertake *essential national health research* (ENHR) to accelerate health action in diverse national and community settings, and to ensure that resources available for the health sector achieve maximum results. Research should not be limited to the health sector, but should also examine the health impact of development in other sectors and the socioeconomic determinants of health which are so important to health promotion and disease prevention. Countries should invest at least 2 percent of national health expenditures to support ENHR studies and a long-term strategy of building and sustaining research capacity.

2. The national efforts of developing countries should be joined together with efforts in industrialized countries in *international partnerships* that mobilize and focus the world's scientific capacity on the highest-priority health problems.

3. Larger and more sustained *financial support for research from international sources* should be mobilized to supplement investments by developing countries. Development assistance agencies should increase their program aid for research and commit at least 5 percent of health project aid for ENHR and research capacity building. External agencies should allow greater latitude to developing-country research institutions by offering more program aid rather than exclusively project support, and by making long-term commitments, for at least 10 years, when embarking on support for institutional capacity building. Special research agencies like the International Development Research Centre of Canada and the Swedish Agency for Research Cooperation with Developing Countries and private foundations should continue to pioneer in health research, and industry should be encouraged to support health research that is relevant both to its own mandate and to the interests of developing countries.

4. Finally, an *international mechanism* should be established to monitor progress and to promote financial and technical support for research on health problems of developing countries.

These recommendations together would, in our judgment, mobilize the power of research to enable developing countries to strengthen health action and to discover new and more effective means to deal with unsolved health problems. They reflect the central fact that wise policy and management decisions in health and development depend on the results of research. Research, therefore, is essential in every country, no matter how poor, to guide domestic and foreign investments and to ensure that its unsolved health problems receive attention on the international agenda of research collaboration. Research will strengthen the ability—and the resolve—of developing countries to meet the needs of the most disadvantaged and, reinforced by international scientific and financial resources, to accelerate progress toward the fundamental goal of equity in health.

Part One

THE CHALLENGE

Fig. 1.1 Life expectancy at birth, 1984

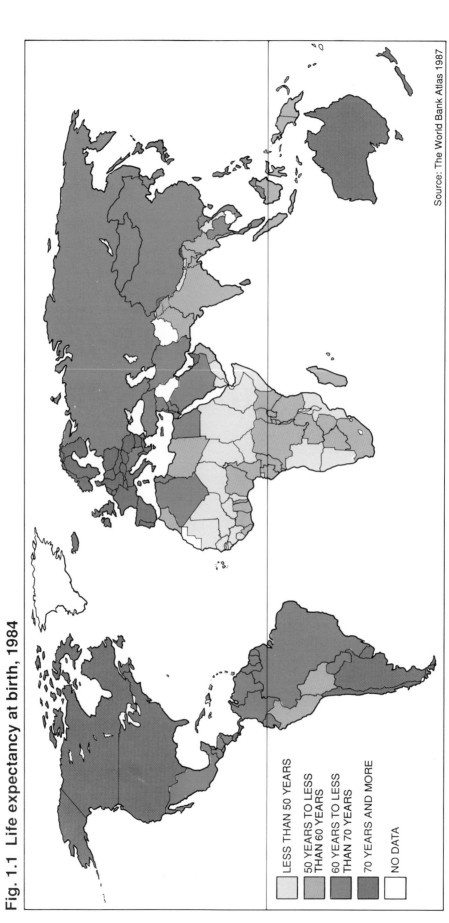

Source: The World Bank Atlas 1987

LESS THAN 50 YEARS

50 YEARS TO LESS
THAN 60 YEARS

60 YEARS TO LESS
THAN 70 YEARS

70 YEARS AND MORE

NO DATA

CHAPTER 1

Health and Development

As the close of this century approaches, the universal goal of "Health for All by the Year 2000" is quietly slipping away. This objective of global health equity was endorsed by the world community at the Alma-Ata Conference on Primary Health Care in 1978.[1] The substantial progress made during the past decade has recently slowed, and in some countries health indicators have actually worsened.[2] To understand what progress has been made, why it has stalled in some places, and what should be done, this chapter reviews current global health status and the relationship between health and development in a changing world.

World Health Disparities

The world health picture presents a distressing contradiction. On the one hand, unprecedented progress has been achieved in this century, more so than in any earlier period of human history. At the beginning of the century, few would have dreamed that today one-fifth of the world's 5 billion people—those in privileged circumstances—would enjoy an average life expectancy approaching 80 years and a lifetime comparatively free of disability. On the other hand, the fruits of progress have not been equitably shared. Many people have been left behind.[3] One-third of the world's people, about 1.6 billion living in the least well-off countries of Africa, Asia, and Latin America, suffer overwhelmingly the world's burden of avoidable illness and premature death (Figure 1.1).

Today's global health disparities are the result of uneven progress in health and development. In industrialized societies health improvements have been underway for well over a century. For most developing societies, however, advances began to accelerate only in the second half of this century.[4] While virtually all developing countries have made some progress, the pace and level of their health gains vary greatly. Figure 1.2 shows the different rates of life expectancy improvements in Ethiopia, Indonesia, and Mexico in comparison to the more favorable experiences of Sweden and Japan.

Every year in the developing world nearly 15 million children die from infection and malnutrition—40,000 children each day or nearly 2,000 every hour. Up to half a million women die from complications associated with pregnancy. Those who survive face repeated onslaughts of disease. Millions suffer from parasitic diseases,

> *On the eve of the twenty-first century, there is great public anxiety about development, environment, and health. At the same time, it has become more and more clear that health goes hand in hand with economic and social development. The questions are how serious is the threat to health, what is to be done about it, and who will do it?*
>
> **Hiroshi Nakajima**
> *Director-General, World Health Organization*

Fig. 1.2 Life expectancy trends (past and projected) in five countries

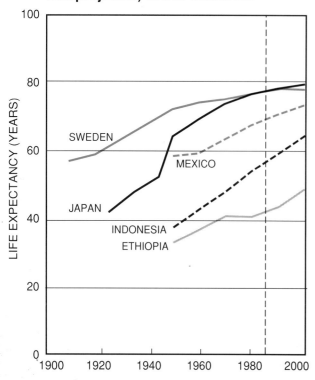

Sources: UN World Population Prospects 1986
Ministry of Health and Welfare, Japan 1987

injury, blindness, and serious disabilities of many kinds. Although less dramatic than death, the burden of illness in childhood and the productive years of adult life causes much suffering and hampers socioeconomic development.

Good and bad health circumstances are not exclusively demarcated by national boundaries. A health continuum exists worldwide—between and within nations. Disadvantaged groups in rich countries are often in worse health than better-off groups living in poor countries. In some developing countries, an increasingly affluent middle class enjoys health conditions approaching those of industrialized countries.

For example, the health prospects of a girl born to a landless farm family in a rural area of the Indian state of Bihar are far bleaker than those of a boy born of an urban middle-class family in the Indian state of Kerala. The mortality risk in the first year of life of a black baby born in the United States is twice that of an American white baby. Figure 1.3 illustrates differences in infant survival both across and within countries. A similar continuum is noteworthy among adults. Japanese men have an 11 percent chance of dying between ages 15 and 60. For white American men, that same probability is 18 percent. For black American men, however, the chance of dying between ages 15 and 60 is 30 percent, a level comparable to that experienced by men in sub-Saharan Africa.[5]

Changing Contexts

These disparities reflect stark inequities in global health and development. The world community has the resources to ensure that the fruits of health progress are shared more equitably by all of humankind. In reality, though, health attainment within and between nations has fallen tragically short of this promise.

Meeting this challenge requires an understanding of the dynamic transition in health taking place around the world: the evolving epidemiological pattern of disease, the obstacles impeding health action, the impact of economic recession, and the longer-term problems of rapid population growth and environmental sustainability.

Health transition

Over the course of this century, the historically important infectious diseases have declined to very low levels in industrialized countries.[6] These health problems of poverty and underdevelopment have been replaced by chronic and degenerative diseases of adult life, such as cancer, stroke, lung and heart disease, arthritis, and impairment of the nervous system. These health problems progressively limit physical mobility, mental functioning, and independent living.

Among developing countries, the pace and direction of the epidemiological transition vary considerably. For many, the transition has barely begun. An unfinished agenda of pre-transitional health problems—infectious and parasitic disease, nutritional deficiencies, and reproductive health problems—still causes a substantial share of deaths in the Third World. Infectious diseases, for example, account for less than 10 percent of deaths in industrialized countries but over one-third of all deaths in the developing world, where life expectancy is still low (Figure 1.4).

At the same time, many developing countries, as they improve health and life expectancy and reduce fertility, are facing a growing burden of chronic and degenerative diseases, usually considered industrialized-country problems.[7] Moreover, the devastating global AIDS pandemic underscores the emergence of new health threats, such as the worldwide propagation of addictive substances (tobacco, alcohol, and addictive drugs), occupational hazards, and environmental contamination. These new threats are often experienced in common by both developing and industrialized societies.

Fig. 1.3 Infant mortality rate in selected populations

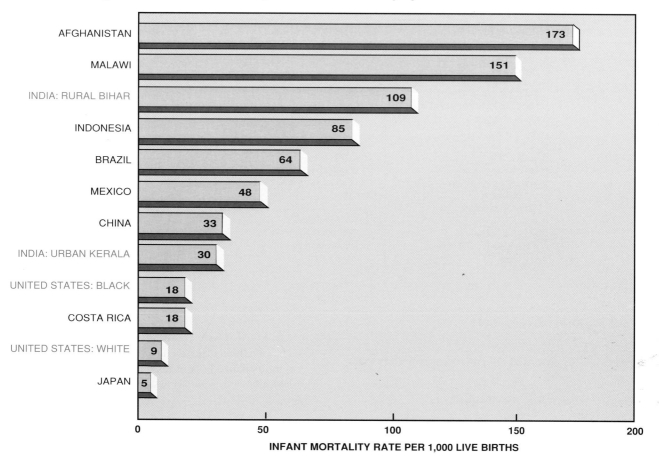

Sources: UN Population Division 1987, Ministry of Health, India 1987, Children's Defense Fund 1989

Many developing countries, therefore, are coping with two stages of the epidemiological transition simultaneously (Table 1.1, page 6). This double burden is straining the capabilities of developing-country health systems. The resulting pressures may stall progress and further widen health disparities.

Health action

The 1980s witnessed the launching of many national and international health initiatives following the WHO-sponsored Health for All proclamation at Alma-Ata in 1978 (Box 1.1, page 6). Primary health care programs to provide accessible, affordable, and effective basic health services for disadvantaged populations were expanded throughout the developing world. One example is UNICEF's child survival and development revolution, which focuses on the mass dissemination of low-cost technologies through social mobilization and marketing. Many countries have made impressive progress toward universal immunization of children against vaccine-preventable diseases and mass dissemination of oral rehy-

Fig. 1.4 Estimated percentage distribution of death by major causes in relation to life expectancy

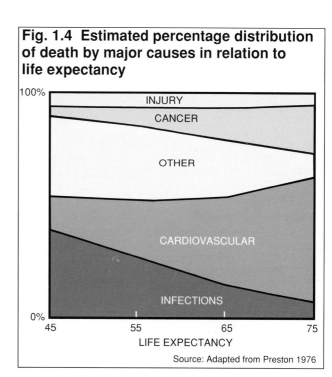

Source: Adapted from Preston 1976

Table 1.1 Illustrative health problems of the two phases of the epidemiological transition

AGE CATEGORY	PRE-TRANSITION	POST-TRANSITION
CHILDREN	Diarrhea Acute respiratory infections Intestinal helminths Micronutrient deficiency Undernutrition Malaria	Congenital defects Growth failure Injury Mental development AIDS Environmental risks

ADULTS	Tuberculosis
	Malaria
	Sexually transmitted
	   diseases
	Chronic parasites
	Injury
	Maternity-related
	   problems
		Neurological/psychiatric
		   illnesses
		Cardiovascular disease
		Cancer
		Injury
		Pulmonary disease
		Eye and ear impairment
		Diabetes/metabolic
		   disorders
		AIDS
		Environmental risks
		Substance abuse

Source: Adapted from Mosley et al. 1989

dration therapy against watery diarrhea. Another example is the safe motherhood initiative, which focuses on preventing maternal mortality by providing family planning and maternity-related health services.

Accompanying these more focused initiatives has been unprecedented growth worldwide of private clinical and hospital-based medical services. These Western medical practices are flourishing, growing parallel with and often displacing a diversity of traditional schools of medicine. The demand for curative health care is driving up health care costs everywhere.[8] Growing demand is being accompanied by increasing pluralism in systems of health care—public and private, preventive and curative, hospital

---

Box 1.1 A decade of primary health care

The international conference on primary health care (PHC) at Alma-Ata sponsored by WHO and UNICEF in 1978 marked a milestone in international public health. At the conference, representatives of 134 governments articulated a historic consensus on the world goal of Health for All (HFA) by the year 2000. Ten years later in 1988, at the midpoint between Alma-Ata and the next century, WHO sponsored a follow-up meeting at Riga. The Riga meeting reviewed the progress achieved and the problems encountered in pursuing PHC. The Riga participants concluded that the PHC concept "had made strong positive contributions to the health and well-being of people in all nations and that the remaining problems called for increased political commitment including making permanent the principles and spirit of health for all."

PHC is an equity-oriented health and development strategy focusing priority on the most appropriate health interventions for the most common health problems in communities of greatest need. The decade of the 1980s witnessed the emergence of PHC initiatives of many kinds:

• Community-based health actions being pursued by diverse private agencies were recognized and supported as PHC efforts advancing the goals of HFA.

• Many governments in both developing and industrialized nations adopted PHC strategies in their health sectors.

• The World Health Organization itself promoted HFA objectives and PHC initiatives within its internal programs as well as with member governments.

• UNICEF launched a "child survival and development revolution," using social mobilization to disseminate low-cost yet effective health technologies for child survival, including universal childhood immunization, mass utilization of oral re-

hydration and the "Bamako Initiative" to provide essential drugs in Africa.

• Several international PHC-related initiatives were launched under multiple-UN-agency sponsorship, including Safe Motherhood against maternal mortality; Better Maternal-Child Health through Family Planning; and a Task Force for Child Survival.

• These actions were accompanied by increased investments by some governments and development assistance agencies in PHC. Furthermore, research was stimulated on the determinants of health, "comprehensive" versus "selective" approaches to PHC, and improved management and operations. There was also a broadening of participation by social and biomedical scientists in the health field.

After a decade of experience with PHC and with a decade remaining to attain the universal goal of HFA, what has thus far been learned? Although a consensus has not yet emerged nor are sufficient data available, there is little doubt that HFA is a worthy goal that has stimulated much debate and action or that substantial health progress has been achieved in many places (for example, in the coverage of children with basic immunizations). Unfortunately, for many, health progress has stagnated or even reversed. Equally noteworthy is the growing recognition of the political, economic, and social dimensions of health advancement (witness the effects of the unexpected emergence of economic recession and debt crisis after Alma-Ata) and the essential need for research—to monitor progress, to evaluate performance, to guide experimentation and innovation, and to shed light on the broader socioeconomic and political factors influencing the health status of populations.

and community-based. Many of these systems are being financed by external sources. A central challenge for the 1990s will be to structure health care systems to achieve greater advances and greater equity in health under conditions of constrained resources.

Economic crisis

The 1980s have been disastrous for the economies of the developing world. The worldwide economic recession and the accompanying international debt crisis in developing countries, especially in Africa and Latin America, have slowed or even reversed economic growth in many nations. Unemployment, inflation, and reduced subsidies have lowered purchasing power,

slowing improvements in human welfare (Box 1.2). In some hard-pressed countries, economic adjustment policies have led to substantial cutbacks in government food subsidies and public services, especially in health and other social sectors. In many countries, social services are under severe economic stress, and innovations to achieve greater efficiency, effectiveness, and equity at affordable costs are urgently needed.

Population and sustainable development

Two long-term phenomena will profoundly affect our capacity to manage world health. World population, now at 5 billion, will exceed 6 billion by the turn of the century and may not stabilize before reaching 8 to 10 bil-

---

Box 1.2 Health and economic crisis

The worldwide debt crisis and economic recession of the 1980s have profoundly retarded economic growth in many developing countries. According to the Overseas Development Council, the slowdown has been particularly severe among heavily indebted countries of South and Central America, Asia, and Africa, resulting in an estimated loss of $2 trillion from the projected economic growth that would have occurred had the growth rates of the 1970s continued (see figure). Highly indebted Latin American countries in the 1980s, for example, experienced a 1.7 percent annual decline of GDP in comparison to the 4 percent growth rate of the 1970s. Some African countries have experienced even greater difficulties. Per capita income in Ghana has fallen by 30 percent in nominal terms, and Ghanaian wages have fallen by 80 percent in real terms. Interest payments on international debt have resulted in a net flow of resources from the developing to the industrialized world, beginning in 1984.

While the human cost of the economic crisis is difficult to measure, UNICEF has estimated that the rate of decline in child mortality slowed in the period from 1980 to 1985 in comparison with the rate of decline from 1950 to 1980, altogether resulting in an excess of approximately a quarter of a million child deaths. An increasing prevalence of malnutrition and a reduction in food purchasing power and finances for health care have been reported in many countries.

The mechanisms by which the economic squeeze affects health are straightforward. Lower wages and purchasing power among the poor and middle-class translate into reduced health care expenditures. Increases in food prices and withdrawal of government subsidies reduce essential consumption. Cutbacks in government budgets result in reduced services in the social sectors. In many countries, health sector funds have been cut by 50 percent or more, with a virtual cessation of capital investments in health services. These immediate consequences are of great urgency, but longer-term consequences may be even more profound as economic stringency takes its toll on human and institu-

tional capabilities that require decades to build.

Research is a necessary, though not sufficient, response to the crisis. Documentation and analysis of the nature of the economic crisis and its human consequences are vital for developing socially acceptable and politically supportable national and international policies. Research is also needed to guide and strengthen direct action. Close monitoring of health status, targeted policies to protect the poor, and more cost-effective actions in the health sector are needed, shaped to the specific needs and circumstances of diverse countries.

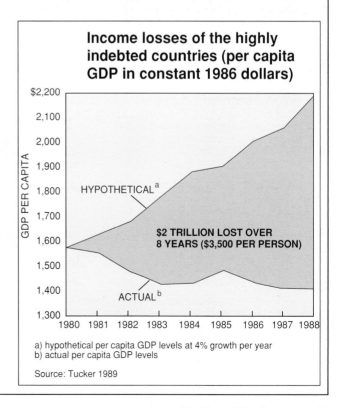

Income losses of the highly indebted countries (per capita GDP in constant 1986 dollars)

HYPOTHETICAL[a]

$2 TRILLION LOST OVER 8 YEARS ($3,500 PER PERSON)

ACTUAL[b]

a) hypothetical per capita GDP levels at 4% growth per year
b) actual per capita GDP levels

Source: Tucker 1989

lion in the next century (Box 1.3). Rapid population growth is generating a more crowded world, hampering efforts to provide education, jobs, and social services, and to stabilize the global environment. Migration to cities is creating an urban world with the growth of mega-cities and an explosive increase in the urban poor and homeless. Declining birth rates and increasing longevity are shaping a more elderly world, with a high-

Box 1.3 Rapid population growth

Sometime in 1987 the world's 5 billionth person was born. Every year another 90 million people are born, more than the entire population of Mexico. By the end of this century the world's population will exceed 6 billion, nearly a fourfold increase since the beginning of the century. This growth both testifies to our ability to improve survival and challenges our ingenuity as we seek to accommodate and nurture such numbers on a fragile and finite natural resource base.

Although the world population growth rate peaked at 2.3 percent and began to decline in the late 1970s, population growth continues to play a major role in development. Demographic momentum built into the youthful age structure of current populations will generate large increases well into the next century—with world population possibly reaching 8 billion by 2020 and over 10 billion by 2100.

Nearly all of this growth will take place in developing countries. The growth will be accompanied by marked increases in the proportions of the population that are urban and elderly (see figures). In 1970 only 25 percent of developing-country populations was urban, but by the turn of the century this figure will reach 40 percent. By the year 2025, 16 of the world's 20 largest cities, each with more than 10 million people, will be situated in the developing world. Accompanying urbanization will be a "graying" of the population in both developing and industrialized countries. A more elderly population will shift the pattern of disease and illness toward chronic and degenerative diseases that are more difficult to manage and more expensive to treat, plac-

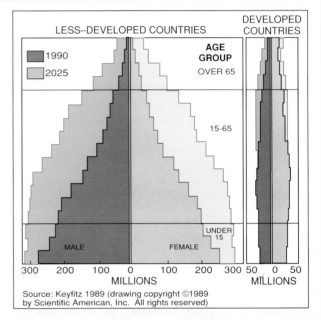

ing great strain on health care resources.

Given these demographic forces, will support of health improvements—generating increased probabilities of child survival and longevity—simply lead to more rapid population growth? The impact of rapid population growth on development is increasingly clear. At the family level, having too many children too closely spaced can set back a family's efforts to improve its own economic and social circumstances. Excessively rapid population growth can also hamper development at the national level. These are reasons to integrate population concerns into national development, but they are not reasons to delay or constrain health advances. On the contrary, family planning and reproductive health care, central components of primary health care, are also key elements of population programs. At any rate of population growth, better health will contribute to greater economic productivity, and improved child survival can influence families' decisions to limit the number of their children.

As Dr. Saburo Okita said in the 1988 Salas Memorial Lecture: "The combination of the following six factors is important in effectively reducing the birth rate: broad-based primary education, an increase in the income level, improved nutrition, a decline in infant mortality, a rise in the social position of women, and decisive governmental action in population policies."

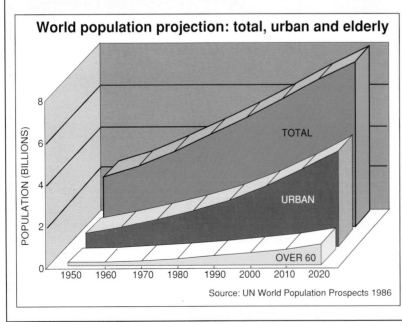

World population projection: total, urban and elderly

Source: UN World Population Prospects 1986

er proportion of older persons in the population. These demographic forces will strain health care systems, especially in the areas of family planning and reproductive health, urban health, and prevention and treatment of the chronic and degenerative diseases of the elderly.

The pattern of development itself will bring new health risks as well as many benefits.[9] The increasingly prominent concept of sustainable development—encouraging equitable economic growth for all today while preserving the basis for future generations to achieve their own development—is highly relevant to the health field. One crucial dimension of sustainable development is equity in health. Slow and inequitable development has already left over 1 billion people without clean drinking water and basic sanitation—the uncompleted environmental health revolution. Yet contemporary modes of industrialization, energy development, and agricultural production that do not incorporate health objectives are generating unprecedented occupational and environmental health hazards (Box 1.4). Schistosomiasis has been aggravated by the construction of dams and irrigation canals, providing breeding sites for the snails that carry the parasite. The spread of Rift Valley fever has been linked to the ecological changes caused by the Aswan High Dam. As in the case of the double burden of disease, developing countries must address simultaneously the dual health challenges of traditional as well as new environmental threats.

Why Act?

For people in industrialized countries, there are compelling reasons to care about the health of people in developing countries—the humanitarian need to overcome gross health inequities, self-interest for self-protection, and mutual learning for joint action. Humanity has entered an era of health interdependence; the shrinking world is becoming a "global health village" with shared health threats, large-scale international movement of people and disease, and an increasing need for joint action. Many of today's health problems—AIDS, population growth, environmental health—are jointly shared and cannot be addressed alone by isolated communities or nations. Health interdependence suggests joint responsibility to address shared problems, for the common benefit of all.

For those in developing countries, health should be given higher priority than is customary because good health is one of the most important objectives of development. People everywhere want to live healthier and longer lives. Development means more than economic growth alone; it means the realization of human potential and the satisfaction of basic human needs. But health

should not be seen simply as an objective of development. What has not been sufficiently recognized is that good health is a positive force driving development. Health is more than a consumer item; investing in health increases the human capital of a society. And, unlike roads and bridges, whose investment value dwindles as they deteriorate over time, the returns on health invest-

---

Box 1.4 Environmental risks and health

In the early hours of December 3, 1984, one of the worst industrial accidents in world history took place in Bhopal, India. Methyl isocyanate from a Union Carbide pesticide plant escaped into the air and caused thousands of deaths and disabilities. An estimated 200,000 people were exposed to the toxic fumes that extended over an area of 40 square kilometers. The ultimate health impact of the Bhopal tragedy may never be fully known.

Environmental hazards are familiar health threats in developing countries. At least 1 billion people still lack access to clean drinking water and adequate sanitation. Compounding these traditional environmental health problems is the emergence of new threats. Air, water, and food chains are deluged with chemical, physical, and biological pollutants. These hazards are increasingly being recognized as major causes of respiratory disease and cancer. These problems are not confined to developing countries alone, as was shown by the nuclear energy accidents at Three Mile Island in the United States and Chernobyl in the Soviet Union. Indeed, environmental issues have rapidly emerged as major concerns of people in industrialized countries faced with air and water pollution, the threat of global warming due to ozone depletion, acid rain, and the hazards of nuclear energy development.

Environmental health problems are often the result of development processes in which industrial, agricultural, and economic objectives are pursued without taking into account possible harmful environmental repercussions, generating unanticipated—and often unprecedented—health risks. Sustainable development, by which today's people can enjoy the fruits of progress equitably without compromising future generations, has emerged as a prominent movement throughout the world. These objectives are important, given that the poor of all nations are frequently at a greater risk of exposure to environmental hazards but have limited access to corrective actions.

While industrialized countries cope with many new threats, developing countries are facing the double challenge of traditional environmental problems and new environmental threats that accompany development. In addition, since many environmental health problems have transnational origins and international consequences, international cooperation, informed and guided by research, will be essential to meet these challenges.

ments can generate high social returns for a lifetime and well into the next generation.

Children who are healthy grow and learn better; sound nutrition improves their cognitive development and school attendance, thereby enhancing their development of skills for employment (Box 1.5). Poor child survival and development waste the assets of a society. Moreover, high death rates among children hinder the behavioral transition from high to low fertility that slows rapid population growth. The productivity of families and nations also depends upon healthy adults. Disabilities such as blindness due to onchocerciasis not only compromise the labor force but increase the ratio of dependents to productive adults. Moreover, the incapacitation or loss of

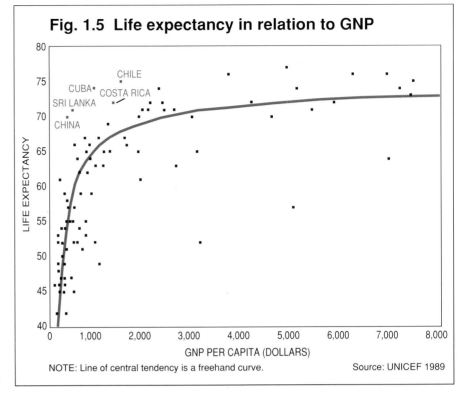

Fig. 1.5 Life expectancy in relation to GNP

NOTE: Line of central tendency is a freehand curve.

Source: UNICEF 1989

Box 1.5 Nutritional strategies to enhance education and productivity

It is estimated that 350–500 million people throughout the developing world are at nutritional risk because they have marginal access to a basic diet. They lack the means to obtain the amounts and kinds of food they ought to have. The resulting chronic shortages of energy and essential nutrients have lasting effects on health and on mental and physical development, effects that impede full economic productivity.

When total food intake is low, the diet does not provide enough energy to maintain both body weight and a moderate level of physical activity. To live, people must adjust their activity within the limits of what they have to eat. Decisions about which tasks adults forego as a means of adapting to chronic food deprivation have profound effects on the well-being of families and communities. Poor households justifiably give priority to tasks seen as critical to survival. The tasks they set aside may be those necessary to the adequate care and nurturance of children, the maintenance of hygienic conditions, or the social interactions that lead to personal development, build community, and give pleasure to life. Adoption of least-risk strategies for survival is a deterrent to innovation.

Children born into conditions of deprivation are likely to be undersized at birth and vulnerable to the combined effects of their mother's deprivation and a disease-ridden environment. Those who survive early childhood grow poorly, never reaching their full genetic potential. Their reduced

muscle mass limits their physical work capacity as adults and, by implication, their productivity in heavy physical labor. Mental development also is impaired in children reared under such conditions. They are less likely to benefit from the limited educational opportunities their environment offers and, barring some effective intervention, are ill-equipped to handle the technological advances that underpin modern economic development.

Anemia, like chronic food deprivation, also reduces work capacity and hampers productivity. It is the most prevalent nutrition-related disease, with an estimated 800–900 million cases worldwide, mainly in the developing countries. Anemia is due to lack of iron or poor absorption of iron in the diet, sometimes coupled with deficiencies of certain B-vitamins and the presence of hookworm and malaria. Intervention studies suggest that as much as a 10–30 percent reduction in productivity can be ascribed to anemia.

Deficiencies of vitamin A and of iodine place additional burdens on productivity. Iodine deficiency (recognizable as goiter) affects the thyroid gland, causing both mental and physical sluggishness. Severe deficiency results in the condition called cretinism, characterized variably by severe mental retardation, dwarfing, and permanent deafness. The numbers of people at risk for moderate iodine deficiency are very large, about 740 million worldwide. Overt cretinism affects about 3.2 million people, half of whom are in Southeast Asia.

Box 1.6 The ratchet effect: a vicious cycle of illness and poverty

An Indian mother of five children, two of whom are now dead, desperately seeks help to save her youngest son. Arriving home after working in the fields, she finds the boy ill with diarrhea. She spends her family's money to obtain help from a local medical practitioner. When the child's condition does not improve, he is taken to a hospital 40 kilometers away; the visit is paid for with money borrowed from a village moneylender. After three days, the boy dies. The woman has not only lost another child, but has spent her money, forfeited four days of wages, and is now in debt.

In the southern Philippines a woman struggles to care for her chronically ill husband and to keep her five children healthy. Several years ago her husband coughed up blood, and a government hospital diagnosed tuberculosis. He initially improved after taking some medicines, but the bloody cough returned. The couple again returned to the hospital, each time spending their available money and borrowing more to feed themselves during the days lost from work. Now, in addition to suffering the ills of poverty, the woman has also begun to cough up blood. She worries about how her five children will be looked after if she and her husband are no longer able to care for them.

Robert Chambers at the Institute for Development Studies in Sussex has coined the term "ratchet effect" to describe this vicious cycle of illness and impoverishment in which emergency health expenditures for a sick family member may lead to more poverty, and may increase vulnerability to illness within an entire household. In this view, the direct and indirect effects of sickness need to be calculated for all household members. Though it is customarily considered a consumer item, good health is essential to a family's economic productivity, particularly among the poor who have few assets to buffer them against the immediate costs of illness and stresses of poverty. When the value of physical labor is diminished, what had been an impoverished but functional family may become vulnerable. The health of adult men and women is especially critical for family survival.

The 15-year history of a family in Guinea in which the head of the household was stricken with river blindness illustrates the social and economic impact of the disease (see figure). A 35-year-old father becomes infested with onchocerciasis (phase 1), and two years later develops visual impairment (phase 2). At age 40 the visual impairment is severe (phase 3), compromising his economic support of the household. Meanwhile, his wife, who recently lost a newborn to measles, develops tuberculosis. Her health deteriorates because, given her husband's disability, and the departure of a married daughter, she must carry more than her normal share of the family work load. By age 42 the father is totally blind, and a 12-year-old daughter also has developed visual impairment (phase 4). Fifteen years after the head of the household contracted the disease, the family is destitute, with two fully blinded members, a wife dead from tuberculosis, and a son who has migrated from the household owing to the inordinate

support required of him (phase 5).

Research on health and poverty not only can advance understanding but can also help more effectively to shape policies and programs. Research on the ratchet effect, for example, has underscored the importance of preventive health services, early curative intervention, the development of innovative forms of insurance among the poor, and maintenance of the health of breadwinners to prevent family impoverishment.

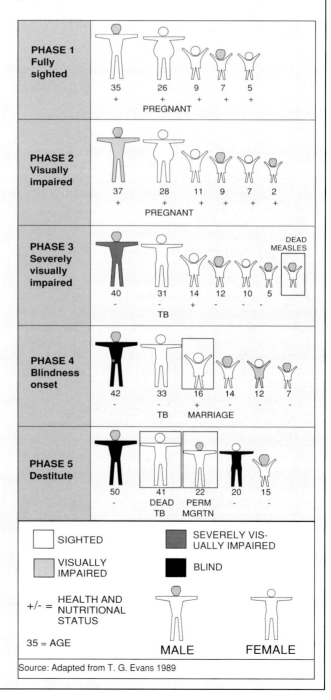

Source: Adapted from T. G. Evans 1989

an adult breadwinner can precipitate a family crisis that triggers a vicious cycle of impoverishment (Box 1.6, page 11). Preventing illness and premature death can thus contribute to the alleviation of mass poverty, overcoming a key obstacle to development.

Paths to Good Health and Development

What are the paths to good health and development? We consider two elements essential: equitable socioeconomic development and enhanced cost-effectiveness of policies and actions in the health sector.

Development for health

National development that emphasizes growth, equity, and sustainability is critical to the health of populations. Conversely, poorly planned development without due regard to health can lead to increased health risks and inequities. The strongly positive relationship between a society's economic performance and its health is well documented. Some societies, however, have been able to achieve far better health outcomes than would be expected at their comparatively low income levels (Figure 1.5, page 10). "Good health at low cost" has been achieved through many factors, including political commitment to equitable development, widespread primary education and literacy, enhanced status and opportunity for women, accessible health services, and strong public consciousness over health rights. These welfare advances have been attained in countries as diverse as Sri Lanka, China, Chile, Cuba, and Costa Rica—across a wide spectrum of political ideologies and social, cultural, and historical circumstances.

Health policies and health action

The health sector possesses many instruments for advancing health that have been neither sufficiently developed nor effectively applied. It is insufficiently recognized, for example, that the primary role in achieving good health is played by the individual and the family. Dissemination of health information can empower people to improve health practices, change lifestyle, or use health services more effectively. The success of personal actions, however, depends upon a facilitating environment shaped by socioeconomic development as well as specific health actions, especially access to effective health services at affordable cost.

The Value of Research

In the end, two tasks are fundamental. First, developing countries must be able to apply effectively what is already known. A substantial share of the unnecessary illness and early deaths in the developing world can be prevented, treated, or alleviated by sound policies and action using strategies and technologies that already exist. Successful application, however, depends upon commitment and motivation, leadership and human capabilities, financial and organizational resources. Success also requires a sound knowledge base in order to empower those who would act with the necessary knowledge and tools to achieve their goals. The changing health contexts—the double burden of diseases, the increasing demand for curative health services, and escalating health care costs under conditions of economic stringency—all underscore the need for innovations in order to increase the impact of health action with limited resources. Research is needed to guide and accelerate the application of existing knowledge and technologies in diverse settings around the world.

Second, fresh strategies and new tools are needed to tackle difficult problems for which current knowledge is inadequate. The dynamic shifts taking place in the patterns of disease require a capability to monitor change and target interventions for the highest priority problems. Just as oral rehydration therapy for watery diarrheas came from research undertaken in South Asia only 20 years ago, and ivermectin, a drug for river blindness, came from industrial research in the past two decades, research is urgently needed on a worldwide basis to find better and lower-cost means for dealing with many health problems for which existing knowledge does not provide effective solutions. Our knowledge and instruments to deal with many old problems (e.g., malaria) and new ones (e.g., AIDS, substance abuse, environmental health hazards) are simply inadequate. Research is needed to develop approaches that will sustain health progress and overcome health disparities.

We, of course, do not argue that research alone will solve all problems. Commitment, resources, and management are fundamental to success. What we do argue is that health research is just as essential—essential to facilitate health action within communities and nations, and essential to generate new knowledge worldwide. Few believe that research is unimportant, but many believe that it is for tomorrow or only for the affluent nations. We believe that research is essential today and is critical for those who must accomplish more with less. This book is about how to realize the promise of research for health and development.

CHAPTER 2

Why Research?

research is a systematic process for generating new knowledge. A Nigerian farmer planting two kinds of sorghum side by side to compare yields, a French biochemist sequencing the proteins of a new virus, a Jamaican statistician analyzing the health impact of an intervention over space and time, a Pakistani sociologist questioning villagers about their feelings toward family planning—all are doing research, whether the instrument is an electron microscope, hospital records, a microcomputer, or a pencil and paper.[1]

The results of research are also used by many. An Indian drinking clean water from a new tubewell, an American jogging for cardiovascular fitness, a district health manager using information to support field workers more efficiently, a hard-pressed health minister juggling competing demands on this year's budget, the program officer of an international agency seeking to optimize the impact of official development assistance—all are benefiting from the results of research. There is hardly a health-related action in everyday life that does not depend upon previous research.

This chapter discusses health research—what it is, why it is important, and how it can be used to advance health and development.

Health Research Defined

Our definition of health research—the generation of new knowledge using the scientific method to identify and deal with health problems—is deliberately broad. The knowledge sought can be applicable worldwide, as in the development of a new vaccine to prevent disease, or locally, as in the identification of particular species of mosquitoes or of health behavior in a village. Knowledge, both generalizable worldwide and locally specific, is essential to effective action for health. Worldwide knowledge is the basis on which new tools, strategies, and approaches are devised that are applicable to health problems facing many countries. Local knowledge, specific to the particular circumstances of each country (and often of each community) can inform decisions regarding which health problems are important, what measures should be applied, and how to obtain the greatest health benefit from existing tools and limited resources. Thus, in our view, health research is both global and local in nature.

Health research serves four main purposes: (1) to identify and set priorities among health problems; (2) to guide and accelerate application of knowledge to

> *Science and technology ... are a shared heritage of all mankind. East and West, South and North have all equally participated in their creation in the past as, we hope, they will in the future—the joint endeavor in Science becoming one of the unifying forces among the diverse peoples on this globe.*
>
> **Abdus Salam**
> *Nobel laureate in physics*

solving health problems; (3) to develop new tools and fresh strategies; and (4) to advance basic understanding and the frontiers of knowledge.

Health research spans many disciplines, including the medical, biological, social, and management sciences. Health status is influenced by socioeconomic factors such as education, behavior, income, and employment, as well as biological factors such as genetic endowment and disease pathogens. Hence, health research requires the scientific capabilities of many relevant fields—molecular biology, genetics, economics, anthropology, and management, among others.

Moreover, health research in our view is not limited to studies undertaken only by trained scientists. We argue strongly that the talents of a great many more trained scientists than are now devoted to this work would be beneficial. But health research also can be pursued by a broad range of people using the scientific method. Valid and significant health research can be conducted by governmental and nongovernmental agency staff, district health managers, and even the communities under study themselves, as is the case in participatory research.[2]

In summary, then, the purpose of health research, whether it is done by village health workers or by molecular biologists, is to generate new knowledge. The research is performed by testing hypotheses, carrying out experiments, analyzing information, and drawing conclusions. The research may produce a fresh understanding of human biology or the mechanism of disease; it may develop new tools such as vaccines or procedures for case management; it may generate information on a community's major health problems, who is at risk, and how available tools and strategies can best be applied in diverse circumstances around the world. Whatever form health research takes, its value can be judged by two basic criteria: its scientific validity and the contribution it makes to improving health.

Why Research is Important

Knowledge is power, and research is essential for advancing health and development, for at least four reasons.

Action and research

Research is essential for guiding action. While research cannot substitute for action, action without tools and intelligence can be ineffective and wasteful of resources. Appropriate research can inform and accelerate the efficiency and effectiveness of action for health.

Research generates information and understanding that can enable individuals, families, and communities to achieve better health. In industrialized countries, sub-

---

Box 2.1 Smoking and health: a Chinese epidemic

Smoking is perhaps the single most important cause of chronic disease in the world. Of the 11 million deaths in industrialized countries each year, 1.5 million are caused by smoking. The spread of smoking from industrialized to developing countries has reached epidemic proportions. China's cigarette consumption, for example, is already the world's largest. In 1987 an estimated 1,400 billion cigarettes—28 percent of the world's total—were consumed by the Chinese. In China, an estimated 227 million men and 24 million women smoke, each consuming an average of 15 cigarettes per day. If present smoking patterns persist into the twenty-first century, China will have about 2 million tobacco-related deaths per year, accounting for approximately one-sixth of all Chinese deaths in the next century.

The health danger that smoking presents for the Chinese people is accompanied by the certainty of much higher health care costs for relatively ineffective palliative treatment against the cancers and cardiovascular and pulmonary diseases associated with cigarette smoking. If these economic pressures compete with public funding for primary prevention against other diseases, the tragedy of China's tobacco use will be further compounded.

China is not unique; populations in many other developing countries, and women in the industrialized world, are increasing their tobacco consumption. Among the contributing factors are aggressive marketing by transnational tobacco companies and the income tobacco sales represent to farmers and governments. Information on the health effects of smoking has only begun to be disseminated in China and elsewhere in the developing world. Lack of information, plus the deceptively long latency period between smoking and the onset of disease, have blunted the perceived need for urgent response. Today's mortality and morbidity from smoking is only the beginning of the smoking-attributable diseases that are certain to occur in the future.

Our knowledge of the linkages between smoking and disease comes from epidemiological research. Its validity is so overwhelming that action based on such research is indicated even before the precise biomedical mechanisms responsible for the relationship are completely elucidated. Clear understanding of the long-term dynamics of smoking risks and public consensus about the importance of early primary prevention constitute the main line of defense against smoking. This defense requires smoking prevalence and epidemiological information, reforms in medical school curricula, and active health education programs involving the mass media, nongovernmental organizations, and strong political leadership.

stantial health improvements have resulted from changes in lifestyle, diet, and activity. Similar advances are feasible in many developing countries as research yields knowledge about health risk factors, how to make health services available, and other essential infor-

mation. Epidemiological studies on the risk of cigarette smoking, even before the precise biological mechanisms linking exposure to disease are fully elucidated, illustrate the power of research in health promotion (Box 2.1).

Box 2.2 Social action in Bangladesh

Can a private nongovernmental organization (NGO) introduce innovations at the national level beyond the coverage of a pilot project? Can research advance the effectiveness of social action? The answers to these questions are well illustrated by the oral rehydration and tuberculosis programs of the Bangladesh Rural Advancement Committee (BRAC), an NGO committed to alleviating poverty among Bangladesh's most disadvantaged people, the 50 million landless poor.

Begun in 1980, the BRAC Oral Therapy Extension Program (OTEP) has reached nearly 12 million households. OTEP uses a system of health education visits by trained village women to teach at least one woman per household how to combat diarrhea by producing and administering a "labon-gur" (salt and homemade sugar) oral rehydration solution. BRAC's remarkable coverage was attained by sound program management and operationally-oriented field research. BRAC's internal and independent research and evaluation division helped to establish systematic methods of program design, monitoring, and evaluation. Field research, for example, guided the shaping of a payment schedule for field workers by which their salaries were predicated on the successful completion of their work objectives—the retention of health education by women as confirmed by independent field checks after the education visits were completed. Action research revealed that group teaching of mothers is as effective as one-on-one teaching but at only half the cost. Anthropological research revealed local perceptions about diarrhea, thereby ensuring dissemination of appropriate, credible health messages.

Begun in 1984, BRAC's TB Program was launched in 50 villages in rural Manikganj subdistrict. Undertaken in col-

laboration with the National Anti-Tuberculosis Association of Bangladesh, the tuberculosis program was implemented by briefly trained shastha shebikas or village health workers who identified and treated all cases of TB. Research was critical in overcoming a common problem in TB treatment: many patients stop taking their drugs too soon, before the one-year course of treatment is completed. Few large-scale programs anywhere have been able to achieve effective continuation of 25-50 percent of patients over the extended course of drug treatment.

BRAC met this problem through experimental field research. When TB is diagnosed, patients are requested to deposit Taka 100 (about $3) as a guarantee toward treatment completion. Upon the completion of treatment, patients are returned Taka 75, an incentive to complete the drug regimen, and the remaining Taka 25 is given as compensation to the shastha shebikas. The payment participation rate has been very high despite Bangladesh's poverty. Given the seriousness of TB, BRAC has yet to encounter a client too poor to pay for this life-saving treatment, and loans are available for those without funds. Evaluation research showed that BRAC's TB treatment completion rate is an astounding 92 percent, and shastha shebikas report increasing community receptivity to the program.

BRAC's success is due not only to good management, but also to an independent, internal research and evaluation division. This division, established initially to compile monthly reports about BRAC's field programs, has evolved into a full-fledged research unit with 15 core staff members supported by 70 others, the great majority of whom operate in the field. BRAC commits approximately 5 percent of program resources to research activities.

Box 2.3 Smallpox: the global eradication of a disease

Twelve years ago in Somalia, East Africa, the world witnessed its last case of naturally transmitted smallpox. A decade earlier, member nations of the World Health Organization had resolved to eradicate, for the first time in human history, a major disease.

The successful eradication of smallpox was due to many factors. Political support and international cooperation, led by WHO, were critical ingredients. So too were financial support and good field management. Often forgotten, however, was the role of research.

One key research contribution was the development of a freeze-dried, heat-stable vaccine that made field vaccination in villages without electricity or refrigeration logistically feasible. A second was the bifurcated needle, developed by Wyeth Laboratories, which enabled briefly trained workers to immunize large numbers of people efficiently

and effectively.

In addition to technological advances, operational field research played a pivotal role. The initial strategy was mass vaccination, an attempt to interrupt transmission of the disease by immunizing a high proportion of the population. This strategy was based on the concept of raising "herd immunity" to a level at which transmission ceases. But transmission persisted even where a high proportion of the population had been vaccinated. In 1969 epidemiological research showed that smallpox was spread by close personal contact following a marked cluster pattern around index cases. This research finding formed the basis of a revised strategy. An "identification-containment" strategy of finding active cases, rapidly followed up by cluster vaccination around all identified cases, helped to eradicate smallpox in about a decade.

Box 2.4 Malaria: intractabilty and the need for research

In 1955 WHO launched a plan for the global eradication of malaria based on vector control (indoor spraying with the insecticide DDT) and the use of anti-malarial drugs (chiefly chloroquine) for protection and treatment of infected persons. Today, one-quarter of a century after the World Health Assembly established that goal, the results have been disappointing. Each year, there are 800 million malaria infections and over 1 million malaria deaths worldwide. Currently available tools to combat the disease remain ineffective.

Any malaria control program has to take into account three basic components: people, mosquitoes, and parasites. The parasite invades human red blood cells and has as its transmission vector the anopheline mosquito.

After the introduction of DDT, mosquitoes developed resistance to this cheap and efficient insecticide and also changed their feeding patterns. Some malarial parasites also have developed resistance to chloroquine, and drug-resis-

tant parasites are spreading through many endemic areas. Alternative drugs are few, and their widespread use may soon induce renewed resistance.

New tools and strategies are needed to regain lost ground in efforts to control malaria. Fresh strategies must conserve drugs and pesticides. Conventional diagnostic methods are tedious and labor-intensive and require trained personnel. New diagnostic methods are needed not only to improve diagnosis but to detect resistance. Product development is a slow process, taking nearly a decade to complete.

Research is thus essential in every area: to develop new assays for use in the field that are cheap, simple, and have a long shelf life; to develop, if possible, an effective vaccine; to increase our knowledge of drug and insecticide resistance mechanisms; and to find intervention methods by which local communities can achieve greater control over the disease in diverse circumstances around the world.

Health policies and actions by governmental and private agencies in diverse settings can be strengthened through research. The strategies of primary health care, child survival, family planning, and nutrition programs all use the results generated by previous research investments. Even when appropriate and effective technologies have been developed in laboratories and tested in the field, application research is invariably necessary to apply them in diverse real-world circumstances. Locally specific research is necessary because intervention mod-

els cannot be transferred automatically from one location to another. Examples of locally specific research are field studies by the Bangladesh Rural Advancement Committee to encourage mothers to use oral rehydration and to raise the percentage of tuberculosis patients completing drug treatment (Box 2.2, page 15).

Developing new tools

The potential for health has been transformed in this century by the development of extraordinarily pow-

---

Box 2.5 AIDS orphans: social policy and action

Tragedy has thrust new responsibilities on a 72-year-old Ugandan woman. Two of her sons died of AIDS, each leaving her with orphaned grandchildren. In one of the families, she has three children between the ages of 1 and 6 years to care for; their mother left to pursue the possibility of remarriage in Tanzania (it is customary in Uganda for children to remain with the paternally related family). In the second family are five more children, the eldest 12 years old; their mother has also moved away, also possibly remarried. The elderly woman needs blankets, bedding, food, and clothing. Even more, she needs rest from the burden of trying to feed the children and the psychological burden of knowing that she cannot provide the school fees that would enable them to avoid ignorance, despondency, and eventually juvenile delinquency.

The woman's village is in Kakuuto County of Rakai District in Uganda. The village has 106 orphans, one out of four children. Recent surveys in Rakai District found 25,000 orphans in a total population of 300,000. The rate of orphanage due to AIDS in this area is believed to be the highest in all of Uganda and portends what can happen elsewhere if the AIDS epidemic increases across the country.

The guardians of the orphans complain of food shortages and inability to pay school fees. They report that

when the orphans fall sick, people automatically assume that they have AIDS and medical help is either not sought or not given. As a result, infant and child mortality is likely to climb. The extended family system is breaking down, stretched beyond limits by adult deaths and the burden of caring for orphans.

Village leaders fear famine or starvation among the orphans. They are keen to develop registries to identify orphans, determine the scope of the problem, and monitor the impact of AIDS on family welfare. To government officials and visitors, they suggest vocational training coupled with income-generating projects as part of a village-based self-help project. Essential to managing the AIDS epidemic is the planning and monitoring of social support and care-giving systems for AIDS victims and their families.

Under these circumstances, the AIDS research agenda is more than simply the development of new drugs or vaccines to prevent disease. While it is critical to progress, technological development must be accompanied by social research—to identify the scope and nature of the problem, to plan, design, monitor, and assess educational and other preventive measures, and to develop social programs to counsel AIDS victims and to support their immediate families, including orphans.

Box 2.6 Recombinant DNA technology

Recombinant DNA technology offers immense possibilities for basic investigation of the genetic mechanisms that regulate life. In addition, this technology is leading to practical applications in fields as diverse as clinical medicine (diagnostics, vaccines, and recombinant protein drugs), public health (epidemiological tools), and agriculture (genetically engineered crops).

Recombinant DNA technology involves the isolation of a fragment of DNA (a gene or a portion of a gene) which contains the information of interest and the insertion of that fragment of DNA into the DNA of a vector such as a bacterial plasmid or a bacteriophage chromosome. This recombinant DNA molecule can be introduced into a suitable host cell such as a bacterium, a fungus, or a mammalian cell. Depending on the vector chosen and the particular vector-host combination, the foreign DNA can be integrated into the host's own genome or can remain as an extrachromosomal element. When the genome or the extrachromosomal element is stimulated to replicate, multiple identical copies (or clones) of the inserted foreign DNA will be made. Bacterial extrachromosomal elements provide a very efficient means of generating large amounts of a particular DNA sequence. This technology has several implications. Milligram quantities of a chosen DNA sequence can be generated for analytical or other uses. Alternatively, if the foreign DNA is a coding gene and is inserted into the appropriate vector, the genetic information can be expressed in the host cell, and large quantities of the protein encoded by the DNA can be produced.

The significance of recombinant DNA technology can be appraised by describing several of its applications:

• Pharmacological applications of recombinant proteins include large-scale production of human insulin, clotting factor VIII, and various growth and immunoregulatory molecules. Several of these genetically engineered molecules are being tested in clinical trials, and selected examples are currently on the market.

• Vaccine applications of recombinant proteins include genetically engineered antigens that induce protection against a variety of infectious organisms for which vaccines are either not currently available or are expensive to produce (e.g., hepatitis B vaccine). The recombinant antigen could be used directly, or the recombinant organism itself could be injected and allowed to produce the antigen in the human or animal host.

• Recombinant proteins are used as a tool for the discovery or design of novel pharmaceuticals. Receptor proteins which are targets for hormones or other factors can be produced in sufficient amounts to permit the derivation of novel drugs through design or through traditional pharmacological screening techniques.

• Recombinant DNA itself may be used as a diagnostic reagent to identify genetic material in biological specimens, bacteria, viruses, and parasites. An extension of this technology can be used to "fingerprint" an individual genetically and hence is potentially useful in forensic applications.

• DNA may be used as a probe to map defective genes. This can lead to a better understanding of the molecular defects responsible for genetic diseases and can permit prenatal diagnosis of genetic defects.

• Genes may be inserted in agricultural crops to improve resistance to environmental conditions and pathogens and to increase yields.

• Recombinant proteins with industrial application can be synthesized (e.g., inexpensive manufacture of hydrolytic enzymes with application to the food industry or detergent manufacturers).

Research involving recombinant DNA technology thus offers an excellent opportunity to better understand the genetic control mechanisms in humans, animals, parasites, and microorganisms and to develop new and more effective approaches to the diagnosis, treatment, and prevention of disease.

---

erful tools against disease. A century ago, this generation's grandparents, facing a life expectancy of less than 50 years, could not have imagined the remarkable advances ahead—vaccines to prevent disease, pesticides to control disease vectors, drugs to treat disease. A cheap, effective vaccine against polio has made the iron lung superfluous, and the vaccine against smallpox, adapted in freeze-dried form and administered with simple bifurcated needles, made possible one of the great health achievements of contemporary times—the eradication of the disease (Box 2.3, page 15). Research has developed a broad armamentarium of weapons in the war against disease, including not only biomedical advances but also our understanding of disease causation, health behavior, and the economics and management of

health systems.

All societies today have health problems for which new tools are needed. A conspicuous example is malaria (Box 2.4). The disease has become a moving target against which obstacles to current approaches have repeatedly arisen. Malaria parasites and insect vectors have adapted, changed, and thereby evaded the effects of drugs and pesticides. For many of the new health threats, such as AIDS, our knowledge base is seriously inadequate (Box 2.5), even though rapid advances in understanding the biology and epidemiology of AIDS have been made.

Modern science offers exceptional opportunities for advances that can be exploited only through research. Molecular biology, genetics, and immunology hold enormous promise for better understanding the mechanisms of disease and for generating new technologies (Box 2.6, page 17). A range of new vaccines, drugs, and diagnostics against major health problems may be developed based on modern biology (Box 2.7). A billion people need safer and more effective contraceptives. Modern communications and information technologies can improve access to health information, the management of health care systems, and public awareness regarding changes in health behavior and disease prevention.

Saving money and multiplying benefits

A critical reason for health research is to provide the basis for effective planning and the wise use of scarce resources. Research has been repeatedly demonstrated to be a productive investment (Box 2.8). The returns from research can spread far afield from their source, and benefits can be reaped indefinitely into the future. The flow of benefits is customarily considered as coming from advanced laboratories in industrialized countries, but there are many examples of research advances in developing countries generating benefits in industrialized countries, such as the lower-cost ambulatory treatment of tuberculosis or the development of oral re-

hydration for diarrhea, both developed in Asia. Research can reduce costs because new strategies can achieve more with fewer resources. Research can help identify key health problems and thus target limited resources to save more lives. Management research can improve the efficiency of health systems, producing greater yield for the same cost. Research can reveal better ways to finance the recurrent costs of health systems.

Research and the development process

A better understanding of research, a growing capacity to conduct research, and an increasing number of research leaders are all critical parts of the development process. Research informs the attitudes with which people think about themselves and their world. Research fosters a scientific, problem-solving culture. Without research, a society's capacity to address problems, old and new, is diminished. Research is necessary because new problems sometimes develop very quickly and can cause great suffering before we understand them. Research is also necessary to anticipate problems, because in the complex systems that affect health, common sense can sometimes be misleading. For example, food is the obvious cure for hunger, but food aid can weaken price incentives to local farmers, undermine local agri-

---

Box 2.7 The promise of new vaccines

Vaccines are perhaps the most cost-effective preventive health measure available, and the pace of vaccine development is increasing. In the 150 years following Jenner's 1796 discovery of the cowpox vaccine against smallpox, six vaccines were developed—against rabies, diphtheria, tetanus, yellow fever, and tuberculosis. In this century, vaccines helped to eradicate one disease completely (smallpox) and to control in industrialized countries several important childhood diseases such as poliomyelitis and measles. Current advances in genetic engineering techniques have accelerated the rate of vaccine development, promising large savings in lives and costs.

The U.S. National Academy of Sciences' Institute of Medicine (IOM) predicts a growing array of new vaccines (see list). Over the next one to two decades, vaccines are expected to be developed against several of the diarrheal, respiratory, sexually transmitted, and parasitic diseases, as well as arboviruses. Further into the future may be vaccines against other infectious diseases. Infection may play a role in many other problems: low birth weight, juvenile diabetes, cardiovascular disease, and even cancers (e.g.,hepatitis B and hepatoma). All of these problems are potentially preventable by vaccines.

Modern vaccine research uses new genetic engineering techniques to develop compounds that could be nontoxic and efficacious, could induce long-lasting immunity, and eventually could be low in cost. Using these new biotechnology procedures, investigators can disaggregate complex

molecules and pinpoint antigens that will induce specific immunity. The search for new immunization techniques has generated knowledge that is being applied to other health problems as well, including new diagnostic agents, improved food production and processing, veterinary well-being, and environmental cleanup.

Research and development of vaccines is expensive, but the potential benefits are immense. The IOM estimates that research and development costs for a single vaccine exceed $20 million. For instance, the development of the hepatitis B vaccine cost nearly $100 million. Only continued investment in research, including research on effective application and management of vaccine technologies, will ensure that the enormous promise of vaccines is realized.

Vaccines under Development
New

Respiratory Syncytial Virus • Chlamydia •Parainfluenza Virus • AIDS • Rotavirus • Schistosomiasis • E. Coli • Malaria • Cytomegalovirus •Dengue •Hepatitis A • Other Arboviruses • Shigella • Other Diarrheal Organisms • Rheumatic Fever • Herpes Virus • Gonorrhea

Improved

Pneumococcus • Group B Streptococcus • Hemophilus Influenzae • Typhoid • Whooping Cough • Adeno-virus • Cholera • Meningococcus • Tuberculosis • Leprosy

cultural production, and sometimes increase vulnerability to hunger. Insecticides can kill pests, but the massive use of pesticides can increase pest problems and lead to contaminated foods.

Scientists as citizens perform a societal role beyond technology generation. Individuals successfully engaged in research can contribute to high standards of creativity, independence, and commitment to truth. All of these values are part of social and human development.

In summary, research is a system involving people, institutions, and processes (Fig 2.1). Its pursuit depends on systematic analysis, creativity, and exploration. Results from research traverse many channels to find their ultimate use. The social benefits of research, in turn, help to stimulate an effective demand for research.

Research and its demand and use are dependent upon the underlying intellectual and organizational capacity of a society. Research policy deals with research processes, the application of findings, research capacity,

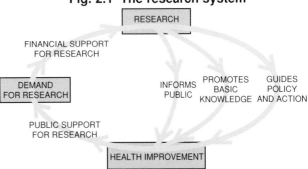

Fig. 2.1 The research system

Box 2.8 The cost-effectiveness of health research

How do we know whether a health research project is a good investment? Successful research generates knowledge that may lead to new technologies (for example, a new vaccine) or to new health care methods (for example, a new strategy for delivering community health services). But novelty is not a sufficient test. The objective of health research is to find ways to attain better health given limited resources of time, facilities, and funds—in economists' language, to achieve more effective health outcomes per unit of cost. A good investment in health research will yield results that are cost-effective when applied in health action.

Rigorous cost-effectiveness analysis is relatively scarce in the health field. Even without it, one can easily cite ways in which research can lead to health improvements and/or lower health costs. Research can find:

• new and more successful intervention technologies and strategies—as the discovery of the polio vaccine displaced the more costly and less effective iron lung;

• less costly inputs to achieve health—as the discovery of oral rehydration solution replaced for nearly all cases of diarrhea much costlier and less accessible intravenous fluids;

• cheaper methods of treatment—as trials in Madras, India, found that ambulatory treatment of tuberculosis was as effective as in-patient management without the higher costs of hospitalization;

• new and more powerful strategies—such as using briefly trained community health workers, backed by a few fully trained health professionals, to extend primary health care to rural villages;

• more efficient ways to deploy resources—such as the practice of identifying and targeting "risk groups" of people who are at greater hazard of a particular health outcome, thereby achieving the largest returns from scarce staff time, equipment, and supplies.

These examples amply demonstrate that health research can yield large and continuing benefits at affordable costs. They support the generalization that health research can be cost-effective, in part because the costs of a successful research investment are finite and limited, while the resulting benefits can yield health improvements indefinitely into the future.

These general conclusions, however, while sufficient for broad qualitative judgments, fall short of full quantitative analysis. The cost-effectiveness of health research is an understudied area, which in part explains low investments in health research. This is undoubtedly a reflection of how recently economists and other social scientists have turned attention to health. By contrast, in the field of agriculture, the returns to research have been studied intensively for more than 30 years. It is important that careful, quantitative cost-effectiveness analysis be used steadily more widely in the health field.

There are methodological difficulties to be faced. For example, in agriculture a convenient measure of comparative benefits exists in the market value of increased output of different crops, but in health it is usually necessary to convert diverse health benefits into a single scale of improved health status, such as years of potential life gained.

Nevertheless, it is plainly possible to make much broader use of cost-effectiveness analysis to support wiser decisions on health research and health action. It is important to move as rapidly as possible in that direction, and it is not necessary to wait while more precise analytical techniques are developed. Good health research is clearly cost-effective. The questions are how much to invest, and how to select the particular lines of research that promise the greatest rewards. A practical guideline in developing countries is to invest sufficiently in health research to be able to obtain optimum health benefits from limited health budgets, and to find less expensive practices than those used in industrialized countries. For most if not all developing countries, this guideline will require a substantial expansion of current health research investments.

and the decision-making processes determining what research is done and how it is supported.

Research Strategy for Health and Development

Essential national health research

From the viewpoint of developing countries, health research is a critical means of empowerment, enabling nations and communities to understand their problems, decide on feasible actions, execute the actions efficiently and effectively, and search for solutions to unresolved problems. Without health research, countries will often be flying blind in their attempts to improve health.

Research may be classified and approached in several ways. For the Commission's purposes, we view two complementary research approaches as essential to the advancement of health in every country. These are research on country-specific and research on global health problems.

Research on country-specific problems addresses health needs, disease profiles, resource allocation, program evaluation, health financing, and other issues concerning the objectives and operations of a country's health system. Such research is the basis for improving national and community decisions on health policy and

> Given limited resources and the immensity of the health problems facing Bangladesh, it is imperative that priorities be set and resources allocated efficiently if we want to have an impact on the health situation of the country. Informed health policy decisions depend crucially on an adequate information and research base.
>
> **Dr. Omar Rahman,** *a researcher from Bangladesh. Remarks at a Commission workshop, Dhaka, Bangladesh, June 1989.*

Box 2.9 Essential research for health in China

A classic use of research for effective national health action was the work of C.C. Chen in Dingxian, rural China, from 1932 to 1938. Through research and experimentation, Chen and his colleagues developed a novel approach to health improvement in China's villages. The spread of the Dingxian model of community health was interrupted by the Sino-Japanese War, but the principles developed there formed part of the foundation for the enormous health gains beginning in 1949 under the People's Republic of China.

A physician trained in medicine and public health, Chen studied with Dr. John Grant of the Beijing Medical College and subsequently became director of rural health for the Mass Education Movement (MEM), a nongovernmental experimental program to improve rural life in China. The MEM believed that China's rural people suffered from four interrelated problems: poverty, ignorance, poor health, and lack of public spirit. The MEM sought innovative ways to promote self-reliance in addressing these problems: an educational system to combat ignorance; the introduction of modern agricultural methods to alleviate poverty; the diffusion of scientific knowledge in medicine and public health to deter illness and disease; and reform in the political system to foster a spirit of public service.

Chen's task was, in his own words, "to devise, through experimentation, a model system affording health protection and modern medical relief to rural Chinese, suitable for adoption in any one of the country's numerous and diverse rural districts." He and his colleagues succeeded brilliantly, finding principles of organization and action that remain valid today:

• They established a basic health information system to identify problems and measure progress.

• They devised an integrated, village-based health services system, with village health workers as the basic personnel, trained, supported, and supervised by persons at the district level.

• The system was designed to fit available economic resources. At first village health workers were volunteers and their services were limited to smallpox vaccinations, education in sanitation, first aid, and referrals; more services could be added as economic resources grew.

• The performance of village health workers was monitored by a strong community organization, responsible for ensuring quality.

Of this innovative health campaign Chen said, "It was economically unfeasible, and would remain so for many decades, for the average village to support a qualified physician or nurse. . . . Yet if we were unable to reach the villages, we would have made little progress in the application of scientific medicine to improve rural health. Our solution, therefore, was to make villagers themselves aware of the problems and arouse their sense of community responsibility and their motivation to work on the problem."

Results of the Dingxian experiment were very promising. Despite the interruptions of war, the ideas developed at Dingxian did not die. In addition to their later use as a basis for effective national health action in China, the Dingxian experiments were among the several important field research projects that strengthened the proposals for primary health care and "Health for All by the Year 2000" at the Alma-Ata Conference.

management by governmental and nongovernmental organizations. It is concerned with improving the effective application of existing knowledge and technologies, as illustrated by the impact of community-based research on health action in China (Box 2.9). Although the methods used for this research are broadly applicable, the results of this type of research are usually location-specific and, therefore, have limited transferability from country to country. Every country, no matter how poor, must carry out this type of research to make the best use of its limited resources. A vivid case for country-specific research is illustrated by the health challenges faced by Mozambique (Box 2.10)

Country-specific research not only guides the wise

> In many countries, health status has worsened in the 1980s. . . . We are therefore under pressure to restore public confidence, and convince politicians that investment in health is worthwhile. . . . But do we have the information to successfully implement our interventions and monitor their impact?. . .
> How do we know that the new strategies will succeed where Health for All has failed? If we do not accompany our new strategies with high-quality research, they will also fail.
>
> **Dr. Jorge Cabral,** *national director of health, Mozambique. From speech at a Commission workshop in Harare, Zimbabwe, August 1989.*

use of internal resources but also strengthens national sovereignty. It places a country in a much stronger position to judge and, if necessary, seek adjustments to external development assistance. Furthermore, it gives each developing country an informed voice in establishing priorities for research on the global scientific agenda. Research in developing countries is therefore essential, not marginal, to the goal of health for all.

Current knowledge and technologies, however, are not adequate to deal with many important health problems. It is also essential that developing countries participate in research to generate new knowledge and technologies for control and prevention of causes of disability and death that occur primarily in developing countries, such as malaria and other tropical parasitic diseases and newly emerging viral infections. In addition, studies of the rapidly growing problems of diabetes, coronary heart desease, hypertension, and cancer in selected populations in developing countries could provide unique insight into the determinants of these chronic diseases and lead to preventive measures of benefit worldwide. The results of this type of research on global health problems are normally transferable

Box 2.10 Essential health research in Mozambique

Mozambique, a country that gained independence from colonial rule in 1975, faces enormous socioeconomic development challenges, greatly exacerbated by war and international forces. With a per capita income of $210 (1986), the country confronts major barriers to achieving its articulated national policy of Health for All. At a Commission workshop in Zimbabwe, Dr. Jorge Cabral, Mozambique's national director of health, stated that: "Faced by shrinking resources for health, we are forced to change the [Health for All] strategy and make difficult decisions about priorities . . . but the information we need to formulate a new strategy is not provided by our present systems." For Mozambique and other Southern African states, Dr. Cabral proposes a "sub-Saharan package" of external support that can meet urgent immediate needs while addressing longer-term national development objectives.

Immediate objectives include reducing infant and maternal mortality, controlling endemic infectious and parasitic diseases, improving basic nutrition, refugee and emergency health, and improving workers' health. Given Mozambique's limited financial, human, and organizational resources, such priority actions can be greatly improved by country-specific information and analysis. What mix of maternity and child health personnel (traditional birth attendants, nurses, surgical technicians and obstetricians) is needed for community-based work and referral facilities? Which are the major endemic diseases and how are they distributed among the population? Are there low-cost approaches to disease control and occupational safety? How can public resources be allocated more efficiently, given the constraint that more than three-quarters of the government's health budget is committed to pay health workers' salaries and to purchase essential drugs? These studies are essential not only to improve the functioning of Mozambique's health system but also to gain the confidence of the public and raise the priority policymakers give to the health sector.

In the longer term, Mozambique must develop its own human and institutional capacity to accelerate and sustain progress in improving health. A critical mass of competent researchers in stable institutions is needed for essential national research. The information and analyses generated are necessary if Mozambique is to adapt its current Health for All strategy to its unique socioeconomic circumstances. Building national research capacity is essential for Mozambique to identify and prioritize its own health problems, to adapt and apply existing technologies, and to optimize the health benefit of limited resources. Enhanced capacity can improve the absorption and utilization of funds, both domestic and foreign, and ensure that Mozambique charts the path of its own national development.

from country to country because they rest on broadly uniform characteristics of human individuals or human societies. Most of the scientists advancing the frontiers of knowledge are currently located in industrialized countries, where working conditions for research are more favorable. In the past, outstanding contributions have come from developing-country scientists. Carlos Chagas of Brazil discovered the parasite and the vector of transmission responsible for the disease that now bears his name. Carlos Finlay of Cuba discovered that the yellow fever virus is transmitted by a mosquito. Today, there are several developing countries with strong scientific capability for health research, and other countries will join their ranks over the next decade as internal and external resources supporting their work improve.

International Health Research Partnerships

To speed up progress on the health problems of developing countries, it is necessary both for the research capacity of developing countries to be expanded and for the research capacity of industrialized countries to remain engaged with Third World health problems, if possible on a larger scale than at present. Furthermore, international partnerships are required to mobilize the

> We in Brazil favor an approach that gives priority to strengthening the institutions we already have. At Oswaldo Cruz we are developing our links with institutions not only in South America but also in Africa. With effort and resources the possibilities to strengthen these ties become very good.
>
> **Dr. Carlos M. Morel,** *vice president for research at the Oswaldo Cruz Foundation. Comments at a Commission workshop, Rio de Janeiro, Brazil, October 1989.*

world's scientific capacity wherever it is located.

International partnerships are being used effectively to strengthen and support research on country-specific health problems. International cooperation for methods development, training and technical advice, and mutual learning from exchanging results, are all highly valuable. Thus research on country-specific problems should not be isolated nationally but should be the subject of lively and stimulating international networks.

Successful international partnerships have also been established for coordinated research on certain global health problems, such as the tropical diseases, di-

---

Box 2.11 Tuberculosis: a neglected disease

Tuberculosis, an ancient killer, remains one of the world's most important killers. There are approximately 7 million new infections and 2.5 million deaths due to tuberculosis every year in the developing world. The burden of tuberculosis is further exacerbated by its age distribution. While children suffer from several forms of the disease (such as tuberculosis meningitis and miliary tuberculosis), more than three-quarters of new cases occur in adults between the ages of 15 and 59—among parents, workers, and leaders. Tuberculosis accounts for one-quarter of all avoidable adult deaths in the developing world. The tremendous toll of tuberculosis will probably increase in many countries, particularly in parts of Africa, due to the interaction of HIV infection and tuberculosis. Individuals infected with HIV have a much greater risk of developing clinical tuberculosis and potentially spreading TB.

The magnitude of the tuberculosis problem is matched only by its relative neglect by the international community. This may in part have been due to false expectations that immunization with the BCG vaccine would solve the problem, or that efficacious drugs (such as isoniazid, thiacotozone, streptomycin, rifampicin, and pyrazinamide) would quickly wipe out the disease. An equally important reason may be the rapid decline of tuberculosis in rich countries, the consequent dwindling of public interest, and the closing of tuberculosis research and training

facilities. Research on this global disease of enormous significance in developing countries has been orphaned by developments in industrialized countries.

For developing countries today, high tuberculosis prevalence and low cure rates urgently require public awareness, political and financial support, and national action—all backed by research. Current action strategies against tuberculosis are among the most cost-effective available against any disease. Operational field research led by WHO and the International Union Against Tuberculosis and Lung Disease (IUATLD) has demonstrated that national tuberculosis control programs can achieve cure rates greater than 80 percent at a cost on the order of $150 per case treated.

To achieve these and even better results, action should be backed by research. Research priorities include improved and simpler diagnostic tests; cheaper, shorter-acting chemotherapeutic drugs; and a more effective long-acting vaccine. Also useful would be research on behavior, particularly drug-taking over an extended treatment course, and research on the design, economics, and management of control programs. These advances can be accelerated through international partnerships that link research to action and strengthen in a coordinated way research activities undertaken in both industrialized and developing countries.

Box 2.12 Substance abuse: a global threat

Of the various addictive substances abused or misused—drugs, alcohol, tobacco—the most pernicious is perhaps addictive drugs. The abuse of drugs (cocaine, heroin, opium, cannabis, barbiturates, sedatives, tranquilizers, and other substances) is recognized as a devastating health problem in many industrialized societies. In addition to adverse health effects on the individual user, substance abuse contributes to profound societal problems, such as family disruption, spouse and child abuse, compromised economic productivity, crime, and violence.

Inadequately appreciated is the fact that drug abuse is a problem common to both industrialized and developing countries—a shared global health threat. A recent study by the Addiction Research Foundation of Canada reported that the highest rates of substance abuse are found in developing countries; out of a total of 152 countries examined, only one of the 14 most highly affected countries was an industrialized nation—the United States. WHO estimates that worldwide there are nearly 5 million cocaine abusers, 29 million cannabis misusers, and about 4 million misusers of barbiturates, sedatives, and tranquilizers. There are signs that drug abuse is increasing in many developing countries, especially those involved in the production and movement of drugs to industrialized countries. Drug abuse in Southeast Asian and Andean countries, for example, has increased sharply, especially among urban youth. Pakistan, with a population of approximately 110 million, reportedly has 1.5 million heroin abusers. There are nearly 2 million opium abusers in the Middle East, Southeast Asia, and the Western Pacific.

Just as the problem of drug abuse is globally shared, so too will international cooperation be vital for effective action. Interdiction of supply must be complemented by reduction of demand and treatment for the afflicted. International cooperation is needed not only to combat the illegal movement of drugs (and the finances associated with the trade) but also to strengthen national and community-level action.

A global effort is also needed to create a comprehensive database and information clearinghouse about the epidemiology of drug abuse and to facilitate interventions to assist both national and international efforts. International partnerships are needed. Priority research topics include experimentation with cost-effective preventive interventions, strategies for identifying and reaching high-risk populations (adolescents, the unemployed, and pregnant women), social and cultural factors associated with abuse in diverse populations, and understanding the economic implications of drug abuse in diverse societies, rich and poor alike. Especially useful would be anthropological studies to determine cultural resources in communities that discourage substance use and facilitate intervention programs.

arrhea, and reproductive health. On the other hand, equally important unresolved health problems can be identified where international collaboration is limited or lacking—e.g., acute respiratory disease, tuberculosis, and substance abuse. While many of the organisms responsible for acute respiratory disease have been identified and some effective interventions are available, more research is needed against this disease—one of the greatest killers of children. For tuberculosis, which is the most common preventable cause of death in adults between the ages of 15 and 59 in developing countries, new methods of case detection, treatment, and prevention must be developed for effective control (Box 2.11). Substance abuse involving tobacco, alcohol, or addictive drugs is a rapidly growing problem worldwide with profound health and socioeconomic consequences (Box 2.12). These are but examples of high-priority health problems which warrant intensive research supported by international partnerships.

Thus we envision a strategy for research on health and development based on the evolution of research capacity in developing countries, linked in ever-strengthening networks of research collaboration with each other as well as with the scientific communities in industrialized countries. All countries gain from mobilizing the world's scientific capacity for addressing country-specific and global health problems. Industrialized countries, also facing health problems many of which they share with developing countries, gain from the new strength and perspectives of growing research communities in developing countries. Both essential national health research and international health research partnerships can result in faster progress for the mutual benefit of all.

Part Two

FINDINGS

INTRODUCTION TO PART TWO

In Part Two, we present our findings about the organization and funding of research for health and development.

Since World War II in the industrialized countries, biomedical and pharmaceutical health research have increased enormously, largely supported by funding from governmental and industrial sectors. More recently, substantial growth has also occurred in health research that uses economics and other social science disciplines to address policy questions. All of these efforts overwhelmingly—though not exclusively—address health problems of industrialized countries. Throughout this period, within the developing countries, a nascent and fragile structure of health research has begun to emerge, varying greatly among countries.

We have observed many organizational, financial, and intellectual links between research efforts in industrialized and developing countries that make it possible for us to speak of an emerging worldwide health research system. In the following chapters, we present several aspects of this system and analyze the gaps and weaknesses within it that call for action.

Chapter 3 examines world financial flows in support of research about health and development. Chapter 4 describes how these resource flows reflect the ways in which priorities for research and action are determined.

Chapter 5 summarizes our findings about health research activities within developing countries, highlighting individual, institutional, and international constraints. Chapter 6 reviews research on health problems of developing countries undertaken by industrialized countries and international centers. The research experience of the agricultural sector, with its international-centers model, is also examined for possible lessons applicable to the health sector.

Chapter 7 reviews the international organizations and programs that promote health research. Finally, Chapter 8 examines the critical issue of how to build and sustain health research capacity of individuals and institutions in developing countries.

CHAPTER 3

Funding Research

This chapter presents our findings on the funding of worldwide research on health problems of developing countries. Our most striking finding is the stark contrast between the global distribution of sickness and death, and the allocation of health research funding (Figure 3.1). An estimated 93 percent of the world's burden of preventable mortality (measured as years of potential life lost) occurs in the developing world.[1] Yet, of the $30 billion global investment in health research in 1986, only 5 percent or $1.6 billion was devoted specifically to health problems of developing countries.[2] For each year of potential life lost in the industrialized world, more than 200 times as much is spent on health research as is spent for each year lost in the developing world.

Of the estimated $30 billion total world expenditure on health research, about $13 billion came from private pharmaceutical companies based in industrialized countries. The remaining $17 billion originated predominantly from governments of industrialized countries.

Figure 3.2 shows the sources of the estimated $1.6 billion of developing-country-oriented health research funds. About $685 million (42 percent of the total) originated in developing countries and $950 million (58 percent) in industrialized countries. Figure 3.3 is a summary diagram of the flow of funds from their source to the research locations where they are spent. A central point illustrated by this diagram is the relatively modest net transfer of research resources from industrialized to developing countries. Out of the total of $950 million in industrialized-country funds devoted to research on developing-country health problems, only $150 million—about one-sixth—was actually transferred to developing countries. The transfer of funds is limited principally because very small amounts of funds from private industry or national research funding bodies go to developing-country researchers and institutions. The major flows to developing countries are from official development assistance, both bilateral and multilateral, and from private foundations.

Thus, our estimates suggest that $835 million is spent in developing countries, of which about $150 million comes from external sources. Another $800 million is spent in industrialized countries on research concerned with developing-country health problems. Overall, therefore, nearly half the research funding on developing-country health problems is used to support industrialized-country researchers working in their own countries.

In spite of all impediments, that goal of sustainable Health for All by the Year 2000 must be pursued. It is the foundation on which national health systems must be built. I believe the financial resources exist in the world to do it, so does the social and political will. We must, however, find a way to harness them such that they act synergistically to achieve the goal.

Olukoye Ransome-Kuti
*Minister of Health,
Nigeria*

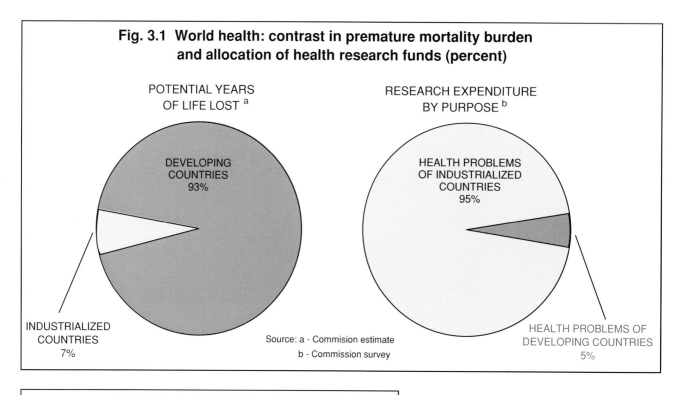

Fig. 3.1 World health: contrast in premature mortality burden and allocation of health research funds (percent)

POTENTIAL YEARS OF LIFE LOST [a]

DEVELOPING COUNTRIES 93%

INDUSTRIALIZED COUNTRIES 7%

RESEARCH EXPENDITURE BY PURPOSE [b]

HEALTH PROBLEMS OF INDUSTRIALIZED COUNTRIES 95%

HEALTH PROBLEMS OF DEVELOPING COUNTRIES 5%

Source: a - Commision estimate
b - Commission survey

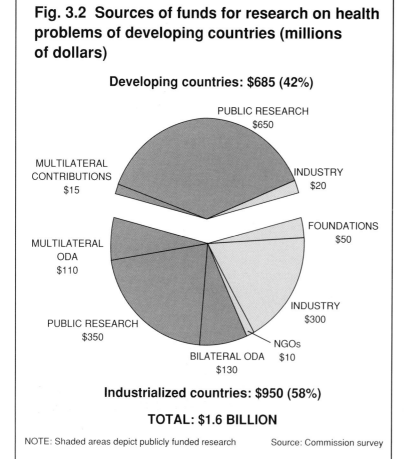

Fig. 3.2 Sources of funds for research on health problems of developing countries (millions of dollars)

Developing countries: $685 (42%)

PUBLIC RESEARCH $650

INDUSTRY $20

MULTILATERAL CONTRIBUTIONS $15

FOUNDATIONS $50

MULTILATERAL ODA $110

INDUSTRY $300

PUBLIC RESEARCH $350

NGOs $10

BILATERAL ODA $130

Industrialized countries: $950 (58%)

TOTAL: $1.6 BILLION

NOTE: Shaded areas depict publicly funded research   Source: Commission survey

The principal elements in these totals and the sources and directions in the flow of funds are summarized in this chapter.

Developing-Country Funding

A major observation is the substantial amount of funds invested by sources within developing countries, overwhelmingly by developing-country governments. Our estimates are based on limited data, and the results should be interpreted with wide confidence intervals. Nevertheless, the estimates show about $650 million of public funds invested in health research directly in developing countries. A very modest additional $15 million is invested indirectly by developing-country governments through their contributions to multilateral organizations such as WHO and the World Bank. Finally, we estimate an additional $20 million was invested for research and development by pharmaceutical companies based in developing countries.

Totals can be misleading, however. Health research funding is highly variable among developing countries. This reflects, in the first place, the uneven distribution of national income. Eight developing countries (Argentina, Brazil, China, India, Mexico, Saudi Arabia, South Korea, and Taiwan) account for approximately three-quarters of the total health research investment made by governments in the developing world; these same countries account for roughly 40 percent of the developing world's GNP. Many countries, particularly the very small and the least developed, invest little or no funding of their own in health research. In these economically pressed countries, research is heavily dependent upon foreign funds.

The uneven distribution of health research among developing countries appears to reflect more than simply the uneven distribution of national income. Our data show that some countries invest more in health research than others at the same income level. The reasons for this are not known, but factors such as a tradition of scientific endeavor and an established and influential research community may be important.

Industrialized-Country Funding

The sources and flow of funds from industrialized countries for research on health problems of developing countries are complex.

Government funds

Funds from the governments of industrialized countries are directed at research on developing-country health problems through three routes:

1. Major public agencies that fund industrialized-country scientists working within their own countries For example, the U.S. National Institutes of Health (NIH) provides very modest support to American scientists working on tropical and infectious diseases. Most industrialized countries in North America, Europe, and Asia follow the same practice of limited support to their own scientists to study health problems specific to developing countries. Total investments of this type in the industrialized countries amounted to about $350 million in 1986. This is a very small proportion (about 2 percent) of total publicly funded health research in industrialized countries. However modest an amount it represents for industrialized countries, these funds constitute a substantial share (about 21 percent) of the research funding available for research on health problems of developing countries.

2. Bilateral foreign assistance agencies that fund research (and research capacity building) intended to contribute to health improvements in developing countries

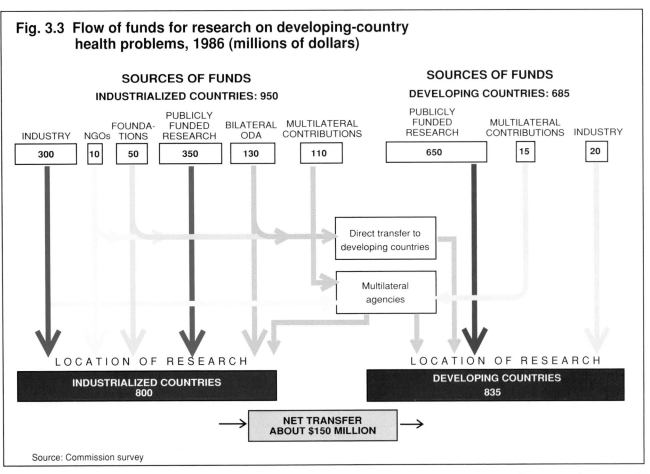

Fig. 3.3 **Flow of funds for research on developing-country health problems, 1986 (millions of dollars)**

Source: Commission survey

Table 3.1 Official development assistance (ODA) for research on developing-country health problems, 1986 (millions of dollars)

| COUNTRY | TOTAL ODA | | BILATERAL ODA | | | | MULTILATERAL ODA | |
| | TOTAL ODA | PERCENT GDP | TOTAL BILATERAL ODA | PERCENT SPENT ON HEALTH | PERCENT SPENT ON AGRI-CULTURE | HEALTH RESEARCH FUNDING | HEALTH RESEARCH FUNDING (VIA SPECIAL HEALTH RESEARCH PROGRAMS) | HEALTH RE-SEARCH FUND-ING (VIA IN-TERNATIONAL ORGS.) |
1	2	3	4	5	6	7	8	9
Australia	752	0.45	513	1.9	10.1	0.4	0.5	–
Austria	197	0.21	141	2.3	3.0	–	–	–
Belgium	549	0.48	362	8.8	11.7	2.0	0.5	–
Canada	1,695	0.46	1,054	2.4	18.8	7.1	2.4	–
Denmark	695	0.84	362	5.7	15.4	0.7	5.9	–
Finland	313	0.44	188	14.3	19.7	0.6	0.2	–
France	5,105	0.70	4,162	4.4	10.1	15.9	0.5	–
Germany	3,831	0.43	2,642	2.1	10.2	2.9	2.2	–
Ireland	62	0.46	25	6.6	18.4	-	-	–
Italy	2,404	0.40	1,487	7.5	13.8	8.2	1.0	–
Japan	5,634	0.29	3,846	3.7	14.2	6.0	0.8	–
Netherlands	1,740	0.99	1,180	4.8	22.2	2.4	1.6	–
New Zealand	75	0.27	61	2.3	20.7	–	–	–
Norway	798	1.15	479	13.8	14.4	2.5	5.5	–
Sweden	1,090	0.83	777	5.7	6.0	4.1	5.6	–
Switzerland	421	0.31	323	3.5	24.5	1.1	2.1	–
United Kingdom	1,749	0.32	1,022	4.3	10.2	6.1	3.0	–
United States	9,564	0.23	7,602	6.9	11.2	70.2	6.5	–
TOTAL	**36,674**	**0.35**	**26,226**	**5.3**	**12.5**	**130.3**	**38.0***	**68.4***

* In addition to the $38 million of multilateral ODA funding of health research via the special programs (TDR, HRP, etc.) shown in column 8, some multilateral ODA funds contributed to international organizations (UNICEF, UNDP, the World Bank, etc.) were allocated by those organizations to health research. In 1986, such allocations are estimated to have totaled $68.4 million, making the total of funding from multilateral ODA $106.4 million.

Sources: Wheeler 1987 (columns 1-6), Commission survey (columns 7-9)

Table 3.2 Pharmaceutical companies: sales and estimated research and development (R&D) expenditures (millions of dollars)

| COMPANY | TOTAL SALES | DRUG SALES | R&D ON DRUGS | RESEARCH AS PERCENTAGE OF DRUG SALES |
1[a]	2	3	4	5
1. Merck & Co.	4,913	4,152	549	13
2. Hoechst	19,960	3,408	473	13
3. Glaxo	3,275	3,275	365	11
4. Ciba-Geigy	10,262	3,045	1,089	35
5. Bayer	20,061	2,874	580	20
6. AHP	4,881	2,840	239	8
7. Takeda	4,248	2,661	269	10
8. Sandoz	5,845	2,662	468	17
9. Eli Lilly	3,537	2,312	452	19
10. Abbott	4,259	2,264	350	15
TOTAL	81,241	29,493	4,834	16

[a] Ten largest companies ranked according to volume of sales of drugs.

Source: Scrip 1988

Bilateral official development assistance (ODA) funds may flow directly to developing-country researchers; they may also flow to industrialized-country scientists doing research on developing-country health problems—usually, although not always, in collaboration with scientists from developing countries. The total of funds allocated in 1986 for bilateral ODA support of developing-country health research was about $130 million (Table 3.1).

3. Contributions to multilateral agencies These are contributions either to specific programs established for health research purposes by multilateral agencies (such as the UNDP/World Bank/WHO Special Programme of Research and Training in Tropical Diseases), or to the general

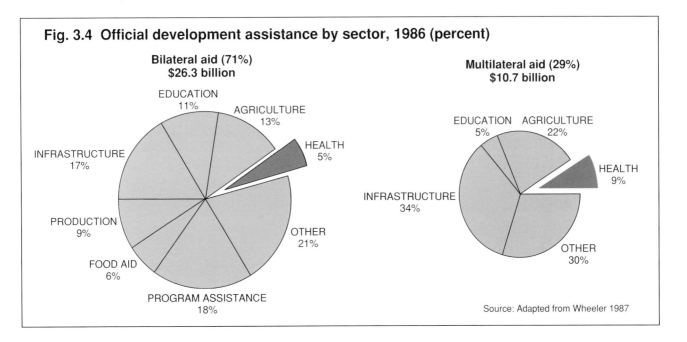

Fig. 3.4 Official development assistance by sector, 1986 (percent)

Bilateral aid (71%)
$26.3 billion

- EDUCATION 11%
- AGRICULTURE 13%
- HEALTH 5%
- INFRASTRUCTURE 17%
- PRODUCTION 9%
- OTHER 21%
- FOOD AID 6%
- PROGRAM ASSISTANCE 18%

Multilateral aid (29%)
$10.7 billion

- EDUCATION 5%
- AGRICULTURE 22%
- HEALTH 9%
- INFRASTRUCTURE 34%
- OTHER 30%

Source: Adapted from Wheeler 1987

budgets of multilateral organizations that allocate part of their funds for health research. In 1986 a total of $110 million went towards research on health problems of developing countries through contributions to multilateral organizations and programs (multilateral ODA).

Both bilateral and multilateral agencies often set aside a small proportion of the funds allocated to health projects and programs to be used for research. The World Bank, for example, includes funds in many project budgets to support planning, monitoring, and evaluation studies that contain research components. Other multilateral and bilateral agencies do the same. In some cases, the funds for planning and evaluation studies come from agencies' internal management budgets rather than their program budgets. These elements of health research funding are difficult to quantify; the estimates reported above capture some but certainly not all such expenditures.

Such research linked to large health projects and programs may yield valuable results. However, the funds often do not contain a research institution building component. Learning from such research usually accrues more to donor agencies than to developing countries, and often much of the actual work is undertaken by foreign consultants rather than national researchers. Because of the size of project and program aid and because their investment usually involves key policy-makers, shaping these very large flows to meet the needs of research and research capacity building in developing countries has high potential for positive impact.

Private funds

Funds from private sources in industrialized coun-

tries are also applied to developing-country health problems through three routes:

1. Pharmaceutical companies based in industrialized countries These companies traditionally invest large sums in research and development (R&D). By our estimates, the 10 largest companies invest about 16 percent of revenue from drug sales in R&D on drugs (Table 3.2), and the industry as a whole invested about $13 billion in 1986. Only a very small share of this large investment, however, is addressed to the health problems of developing countries. Perhaps $300 million may be so directed, principally aimed at new vaccines against malaria and schistosomiasis, anti-parasite drugs, and better insecticides. As well as being small in size, pharmaceutical company research and development addressed to developing-country health problems is conducted mostly in industrialized countries, and research findings are often not easily accessible to all scientists. While this is understandable for commercial reasons, it results in special problems of access for developing-country scientists.

2. Philanthropic foundations These are based primarily in North America, with growing numbers in Europe and Japan. Allocations by major foundations to developing-country health research are shown in Table 3.3 (page 35). These estimates suggest that total foundation contributions to research on developing-country health problems were about $50 million in 1986. These funds were directed partly to supporting research in developing countries, partly as contributions to multilateral programs, and partly to supporting research in industrialized countries.

3. Nongovernmental organizations with headquar-

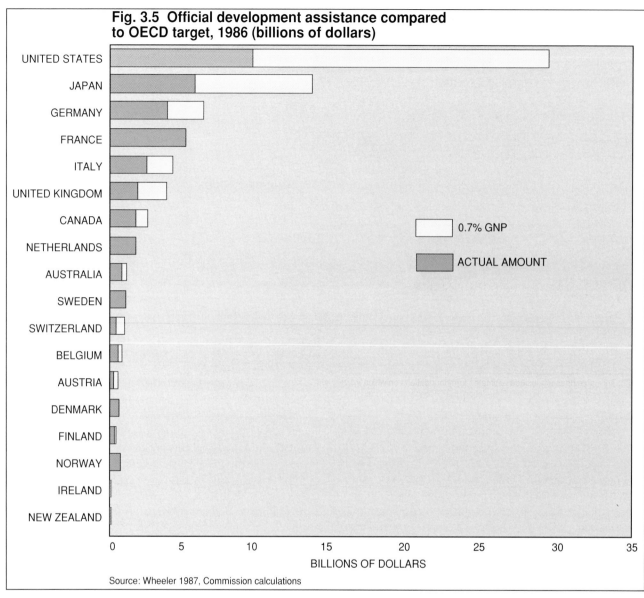

Fig. 3.5 Official development assistance compared to OECD target, 1986 (billions of dollars)

UNITED STATES
JAPAN
GERMANY
FRANCE
ITALY
UNITED KINGDOM
CANADA
NETHERLANDS
AUSTRALIA
SWEDEN
SWITZERLAND
BELGIUM
AUSTRIA
DENMARK
FINLAND
NORWAY
IRELAND
NEW ZEALAND

☐ 0.7% GNP
▨ ACTUAL AMOUNT

0   5   10   15   20   25   30   35
BILLIONS OF DOLLARS

Source: Wheeler 1987, Commission calculations

ters in the industrialized world Many nongovernmental organizations (NGOs), for example Save the Children and Médecins sans Frontières, undertake action programs addressing health problems of developing countries. The NGOs are primarily oriented toward action, not research, and so spend only a small share of their funds on research. Often innovative experimental field actions are undertaken, but they are infrequently analyzed or disseminated broadly. A few agencies, such as the member organizations of the International Federation of Anti-Leprosy Associations, spend larger shares of their funds for research. We have included in our total a rough estimate of $10 million for health research by NGO sources.

The Importance of Official Development Assistance

These data show the significance of development

assistance—both bilateral and multilateral—as the major source of resource transfers for health research in developing countries. The contribution of foundations is also significant although not a large component of total health research funding.

Total official development assistance in 1986 is shown in Figure 3.4 (page 33). Of the $37 billion channeled by 18 countries to ODA in that year (0.35 percent of industrialized-country GNP), about two-thirds was channeled bilaterally and about one-third multilaterally. The percentage of gross domestic product (GDP) spent on total ODA varied widely, from a low of 0.21 percent in Austria and 0.23 percent in the United States to a high of 1.15 percent in Norway. Figure 3.5 shows the additional ODA funds that would have been provided in 1986 if all OECD countries had met their agreed-upon target of 0.7% of GDP.

Table 3.3 Estimates of expenditures on research on developing-country health problems by selected foundations, 1986 (millions of dollars)

NAME 1	TOTAL ASSETS 2	TOTAL EXPENDITURES 3	EXPENDITURES ON HEALTH 4	EXPENDITURES ON RESEARCH ON DEVELOPING-COUNTRY HEALTH PROBLEMS 5	RESEARCH EXPENDITURES AS PERCENTAGE OF HEALTH EXPENDITURES. (COL.5 ÷ COL. 4) 6
Aga Khan Foundation	-	-	-	2.1	-
Carnegie Corporation of New York	715	33.8	3.5	1.1	31
Edna McConnell Clark Foundation	348	18.7	3.4	3.1	91
Ford Foundation	4,759	248.7	10.3	4.0	39
William and Flora Hewlett Foundation	565	164.2	6.1	3.4	56
W. K. Kellogg Foundation	685	96.2	6.7	2.0	30
John D. and Catherine T. MacArthur Foundation	2,271	125.5	11.2	3.5	31
Andrew W. Mellon Foundation	-	72.3	9.2	3.7	40
Pew Charitable Trusts	2,336	133.9	11.9	5.0	42
Rockefeller Foundation	1,615	59.8	18.6	11.6	62
Sasakawa Health Trust Fund	-	-	-	1.4	-
Thrasher Research Fund	23	1.4	1.1	1.1	100
Wellcome Trust	-	-	-	5.1	-
TOTAL	-	-	-	47.1	-

NOTE: This table does not include estimates from foundations on which information was not available, e.g., the Oak Foundation, the Gulbenkian Foundation, etc.

Source: Foundation annual reports

The share of ODA going to health research also varies widely among donor countries. Perhaps the most sensitive indicator of donor commitment to health research is to combine health research funding through bilateral channels and through multilateral health research programs, and calculate the combined total as a percentage of total ODA. Using this indicator, industrialized countries can be divided into three groups:

1) high investors—those that commit more than 0.7 percent of ODA directly to health research: Denmark, Norway, Sweden, Switzerland, and the United States;

2) medium investors—those that commit 0.4-0.7 percent: Belgium, Canada, France, and the United Kingdom; and

3) low investors—those that commit less than 0.4 percent: Australia, Austria, Finland, Germany, Italy, Japan, the Netherlands, and New Zealand.

Though expressed as small percentages, these numbers reflect substantial relative differences. If the countries at the low end of the distribution were to match those at the medium or high end, very large increases in total flows would result[3].

Historical ties and geopolitical considerations, as well as development needs, influence the distribution of ODA from European, North American, and Asian donors. Table 3.4 shows the geographic distribution of the three largest country recipients of bilateral ODA funds from four illustrative countries: France, Japan, Sweden, and the United States. The multilateral programs specifically organized for health research and health research capacity building, such as TDR and HRP, generally apply more direct, science-oriented criteria for allocation, shaped by

Table 3.4 Countries receiving largest percentages of bilateral official development assistance (ODA) from four donor countries, 1985-86

DONOR COUNTRY	TOP THREE RECIPIENTS	PERCENTAGE OF DONOR COUNTRY'S BILATERAL ODA
FRANCE	Réunion	8.5
	Martinique	6.6
	Polynesia	4.5
JAPAN	China	8.2
	Philippines	7.5
	Indonesia	5.8
SWEDEN	Tanzania	8.0
	India	6.3
	Mozambique	5.3
UNITED STATES	Israel	19.1
	Egypt	12.8
	El Salvador	2.8

Source: Adapted from Wheeler 1987

priority research agendas, scientific quality, and capacity-building objectives.

Conclusions

1. Worldwide investment for research on health is estimated to be about $30 billion, but only about 5 percent ($1.6 billion) is devoted to the health problems of developing countries, which account for 93 percent of the years of potential life lost in the world.

2. Developing countries—primarily their governments—invest substantial sums in health research ($685 million, or 42 percent of the $1.6 billion total). Three-quarters of these investments come from eight large or rapidly developing countries. Most developing countries invest little in health research.

3. Industrialized countries contribute 58 percent ($950 million) of the total investment in research on health problems of developing countries. Most of these funds are spent by industry and by public agencies (medical research councils, national institutes of health), for which research on health problems of developing countries constitutes an extremely small proportion of their to-tal research efforts.

4. Industry and public agencies invest their research budgets almost entirely within industrialized countries. The transfer of resources to support health research in developing countries comes primarily from bilateral and multilateral ODA and from foundations. The amount is very modest—perhaps $150 million annually.

5. Although solid data are not available, investment in research on developing-country health problems has probably been static or declining over the past decade due to the economic recession in developing countries and the decline of ODA in real terms.

6. Official development assistance varies greatly among industrialized countries, from 0.2 percent of GNP in the United States and 0.3 percent in Japan to about 1 percent in the Scandinavian countries. Similarly, the percentage of ODA committed to health research varies widely. Modest increases in ODA and in the percentage of ODA committed to health research could generate substantial resources for health research in developing countries.

CHAPTER 4

Research Priorities

*T*he worldwide resource flows described in Chapter 3 support research directed at many health problems and conducted by a wide array of scientists and institutions around the world. Which health problems are receiving research attention? Which problems are comparatively neglected? What are the factors that ought to shape the research agenda, at the national and international levels? These questions are addressed in this chapter.

Health Problems

The major causes of deaths worldwide are shown in Table 4.1. Each year about 49 million people die—about 11 million in industrialized countries and 38 million in developing countries. The best estimates available—necessarily based on incomplete information—show that infectious and parasitic diseases account for about 34 percent of all deaths. Other important causes are cancer, circulatory diseases, perinatal and pregnancy-related problems, and injury.

The major causes of deaths can be differentiated between industrialized and developing countries. Table 4.2 shows the number of deaths due to major causes in the developing world as estimated by three international organizations—WHO, the United Nations Development Programme (UNDP), and this Commission. Because of the uncertainty of the data, the Commission's estimates are shown according to a lower and upper range of values.[1] The causes of death, furthermore, are grouped according to our classification of pre-transitional and post-transitional problems.

In all three estimates, the pre-transitional infectious and parasitic diseases are paramount. Post-transitional problems such as cardiovascular disease and cancer are also significant. Other post-transitional problems—new threats such as AIDS, substance abuse, and occupational health hazards—cause fewer deaths, although their morbidity burdens may be heavy.

As the epidemiological transition evolves, developing countries will increasingly face the double burden of pre- and post-transitional diseases simultaneously. The projected increasing burden of the chronic and degenerative diseases in developing countries between 1985 and 2015 is highlighted in Figure 4.1.

This global picture disguises wide variability among developing countries, as would be expected given their differences in life expectancy, ecological circum-

> *Needs will vary from place to place. . . . In one area, for example, potable water may be a priority issue and in another area, the control of malaria. The safest way to determine those needs is by conducting preliminary surveys. Needs should be identified where they actually emerge, not out of textbooks.*
>
> **C. C. Chen**
> *Professor Emeritus, West China University of Medical Sciences*

Table 4.1 Estimated number of deaths by cause worldwide and in industrialized and developing countries, 1985 (thousands of persons)

CAUSE	WORLD	INDUSTRIALIZED COUNTRIES	DEVELOPING COUNTRIES
INFECTIOUS AND PARASITIC DISEASES	**(17,006)**	**(506)**	**(16,500)**
Acute respiratory infections*	7,768	368	7,400
Diarrheal diseases	5,025	25	5,000
Tuberculosis	2,840	40	2,800
Malaria	1,000	–	1,000
Others	373	73	300
CIRCULATORY, DEGENERATIVE	**(12,430)**	**(5,930)**	**(6,500)**
Ischemic heart disease	–	2,392	–
Cerebrovascular disease	–	1,504	–
Diabetes	–	153	–
Others	–	1,881	–
CANCER	4,793	2,293	2,500
CHRONIC LUNG DISEASE	2,685	385	2,300
PREGNANCY COMPLICATIONS	500	4	496
PERINATAL CONDITIONS	3,300	100	3,200
INJURY AND POISONING	3,172	772	2,400
OTHER CAUSES	5,054	1,054	4,000
ALL CAUSES	**48,945**	**11,045**	**37,896**

* Includes measles, whooping cough, and other related causes of death.

Source: Lopez 1989

Table 4.2 Estimated number of deaths by cause in developing countries (millions of persons)

HEALTH PROBLEM	ESTIMATES		
	UNDP (1988)	WHO (1985)	COMMISSION (1986)
PRE-TRANSITION			
Acute respiratory infections	10.0	7.4	4.2 – 9.2
Diarrheal diseases	4.3	5.0	3.4 – 7.5
Immunizable diseases	3.8	*	1.7 – 4.3
Tuberculosis	0.9	2.8	0.6 – 4.3
Malaria	1.5	1.0	0.4 – 2.0
Other infections	2.6	0.3	0.4 – 1.8
Pregnancy complications	0.5	0.5	0.4 – 0.6
Perinatal conditions	-	3.2	- – -
POST-TRANSITION			
Cardiovascular and metabolic diseases	8.0	6.5	4.5 – 9.9
Cancers	2.0	2.5	1.1 – 2.5
Accidents and violence	2.0	2.4	1.2 – 2.2
AIDS/Sexually transmitted diseases	0.1	-	0.1 – 0.2
Substance abuse	-	-	- – 1.0
Environmental/Occupational hazards	-	-	- – 0.2
OTHER	**2.3**	**6.3**	**–**
TOTAL	**38.0**	**37.9**	**–**

* Not classified; contained in other categories.

Sources: UNDP: adapted from Walsh 1988
WHO: adapted from Lopez 1989
Commission estimates

stances and stages of development. Even within countries, there may be marked variability between regions. In Kenya, for example, malaria is concentrated in tropical lowland regions and scarce in the higher plateau regions. Urban health problems differ from rural health problems. Health problems can also vary between communities.

Even the perception of health problems may differ according to the people consulted.[2] In Table 4.3 the priority health problems in Thailand identified by urban slum dwellers in Bangkok and members of a rural community in Northeast Khon Kaen are compared with those derived from analysis of data by health professionals. The problems are perceived and expressed in entirely different ways by the people affected from how they are seen by the scientists.

Balancing Research Priorities

How well are current research investments addressing the major health problems and meeting priority research needs in developing countries?

One approach to establishing priorities is to relate research investments to mortality data. While estimates of the number of deaths by cause have been made, estimates of investments for problem-specific research are entirely unavailable at the national level, and are only limited and incomplete for international investments. For illustrative purposes, we have made rough calculations showing that funds invested in international programs for research on tropical and parasitic diseases may be on the order of about $20 per year per death, while the same figure for AIDS may be closer to $600. Other problems, such as acute respiratory infections and tuberculosis, receive far smaller investments, only pennies per year per death.

Which groups make international investments, and how are these distributed according to health problems? Our examination of official development assistance in support of health research demonstrates again marked variability. Donor contributions to four major WHO-associated research programs are shown in Table 4.4. Some donors contribute to only one program; others contribute to all four. The rationale for the different decisions by donors is not readily apparent.

The recent explosion of funding for research on AIDS responds to urgent needs recognized in both industrialized and developing countries. There is no doubt of the enormous health significance of AIDS in many developing countries. In one district of Uganda in 1989, blood tests demonstrated that more than half of the

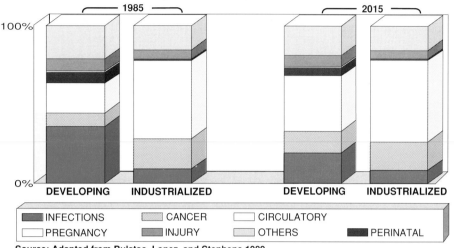

Fig 4.1 Estimated and projected distribution (percent) of the major causes of death in developing and industrialized countries, 1985 and 2015

Source: Adapted from Bulatao, Lopez, and Stephens 1989

Table 4.3 Priority ranking of health problems according to data analysis and people's perceptions in two populations in Thailand

HEALTH PROBLEM	BANGKOK URBAN POOR[a]		KHON KAEN RURAL COMMUNITIES[b]	
	EPIDEMIOLOGICAL SURVEY	PEOPLE'S PERCEPTION	PEOPLE'S PERCEPTION	SECONDARY DATA
1	Infection	Sanitation	Herbal medicine	Matermal/child health
2	Addiction	Flooding	Modern and traditional medicine	Infection
3	Violence	Health services	Prevention/ promotion	Parasite/ malnutrition
4	Young pregnancy	Professional leadership	Simple treatment	Chronic disease
5	Chronic disease	—	—	Chemical/drugs

Sources: [a] Sitthi-Amorn 1989 • [b] Faculty of Medicine, Khon Kaen University 1989

Table 4.4 Donor contributions for selected WHO-associated research programs, 1986-87 biennium (millions of dollars)

DONOR	HRP[a]	OCP[b]	TDR[c]	CDD[d]
Australia	0.2	–	0.7	0.3
Belgium	–	0.6	0.5	–
Canada	–	2.5	2.6	0.4
Denmark	3.6	–	4.6	1.2
Finland	0.3	0.5	0.7	0.7
France	–	1.6	0.8	–
Germany	1.4	1.9	2.7	–
Italy	–	1.2	1.8	0.1
Japan	–	3.1	0.2	0.3
Kuwait	–	2.2	–	–
Netherlands	0.6	4.4	1.8	0.9
Norway	4.4	1.4	5.5	0.3
Saudi Arabia	–	4.0	–	–
Sweden	5.5	–	4.8	1.1
Switzerland	0.3	7.0	2.3	0.9
United Kingdom	5.2	2.1	0.7	0.3
United States	0.2	5.0	5.3	3.2
EEC	–	6.8	–	–
IDRC	0.1	–	0.1	–
MacArthur Foundation	–	–	3.6	–
Rockefeller Foundation	0.7	–	–	–
UNDP	–	2.6	4.7	1.1
UNFPA	5.6	–	–	–
UNICEF	–	–	–	0.8
World Bank	–	5.0	6.1	–
Ciba Geigy	–	–	–	2.6

[a] HRP: Special Programme of Research, Development and Research Training in Human Reproduction

[b] OCP: Onchocerciasis Control Programme

[c] TDR: Special Programme for Research and Training in Tropical Diseases

[d] CDD: Programme for Control of Diarrhoeal Diseases

Source: UNDP/WORLD BANK/WHO 1987

women aged 20 to 30 and 20 percent of the newborns were carrying the AIDS virus.[3] Given such circumstances, it is vital that research on AIDS should have a very high priority. Global investment in research on AIDS in 1988, from both public and private sources, may well have exceeded $2 billion. These very large allocations are primarily driven by forces within industrialized countries, responding to their own concerns about AIDS. Sharply increased AIDS research may also benefit those developing countries that have serious AIDS problems. It is critically important that the research investment on AIDS not divert funds from research urgently needed on other health problems causing far greater mortality and morbidity in many developing countries than AIDS. Some of these problems are of great significance:

• Research on simple and effective treatment of **acute respiratory infections**, one of the most common causes of illness and death in developing countries, particularly in young children.

• Research to improve case detection, ambulatory treatment, and prevention of **tuberculosis**, which remains the most common preventable cause of death in adults during their most productive years in developing countries.

• Research to identify and modify factors responsible for the rapidly rising risk of **diabetes, coronary heart disease, and hypertension** in developing countries, which are not only increasingly important causes of death and disability but also of growing demand on limited resources for health (Box 4.1).

• Research on **fertility and reproductive health** (Box 4.2), which has a continuing claim to high priority for health reasons because unwanted fertility is a major cause of perinatal and pregnancy-related deaths and because infertility from sexually transmitted diseases and other causes may be largely preventable. But there are other reasons that justify making this subject a high research priority: effective contraception helps women control their own lives, helps parents achieve the size of family and spacing of children they can raise with good health and educational opportunities, and helps countries balance the rate of population growth with sound development objectives.

• Research to design and evaluate effective national programs to prevent **micronutrient deficiencies** (vitamin A, iodine, and iron) in view of the profound health consequences of these deficiencies (Box 4.3, page 42). Vitamin A deficiency, for example, is not only a cause of loss of vision, but may also contribute to illness and death in children by making them more vulnerable to diarrhea and respiratory infections.

• Research on problems not classified as diseases, such as the performance and financing of health services, the development of practical health information systems to guide **policy and management** decisions, and methods to reduce the prodigious waste and misuse of modern therapeutic drugs in developing countries (Box 4.4, page 42). Research on traditional medicines and practices is also needed to identify the benefits and complications of these long-established treatments.

Mortality alone is not a sufficient criterion for ranking diseases in order of importance for the purpose of setting research priorities. Health problems that cause much disability but few deaths need to be given appropriate consideration in establishing the research agenda. Giving greater weight to morbidity would certainly move some health problems up the scale of research priorities, for example, mental illness and behavioral problems (Box 4.5, page 43), skin diseases, arthritis, blindness, and deafness. Common problems such as mental illness that are poorly understood are hardly receiving any research attention in developing countries. Similarly, there has

Box 4.1 Are post-transition diseases preventable?

It is conceivable that the Third World might be spared much of the burden of disability and death from diabetes, coronary heart disease, and hypertension that has marked the health transition in industrialized, urban societies. These diseases also account for a large share of health costs in post-transition societies. A commanding priority for global health research, therefore, is the identification and modification of the risk factors responsible for the principal post-transition diseases.

New insight into the powerful interaction of social environment and health, for example, is offered by data on mortality among civil servants in the United Kingdom. The data show a stepwise gradient in mortality from coronary heart disease and other causes such that the higher the grade of employment in the civil service the lower the risk of death. If persons in the lowest of the six grades of the civil service had had the same mortality risk as those in the highest grade, death among those in the lowest grade would have been reduced by two-thirds over a 10-year period. These are startling findings, since persons in even the lowest civil service grade have incomes far above poverty levels; moreover, none of the usual risk factors explain the mortality differentials. Consequently research is underway seeking risk factors linked to social position across the employment gradient, such as working conditions, leisure activities, and lifestyle.

The possibility that social factors may play a part is suggested by the observation that immigrants to the United Kingdom from the Indian subcontinent have the highest mortality rate from coronary heart disease of any population subgroup in the United Kingdom—50 percent higher than average. Field studies have not demonstrated differences in dietary fat consumption or serum cholesterol as an explanation for the excess mortality; the immigrant subgroup did, however, have a high prevalence of diabetes and truncal obesity.

Moreover, the consistency of the gradient in mortality in United Kingdom civil servants from other causes as well as coronary heart disease favors factors which are not disease-specific as the explanation of differences in disease expression. An understanding of coping mechanisms and other non-specific factors at individual, household, workplace, and community levels that influence disease prevalence may be particularly important for developing countries where access to expensive disease treatment is limited by resource constraints.

Box 4.2 Contraception and reproductive health

The promotion of safe and effective contraception is the principal policy tool used by governments to reduce fertility rates and promote reproductive health. Yet, even with recent advances in contraceptive technology, reproductive health remains elusive, in part because existing technologies and delivery systems are inadequate. Worldwide, 500 million people lack access to safe and effective fertility regulation. Each year 30–55 million induced abortions take place due to lack of access to high quality contraception, method failure, and insufficient information and education on sexuality and reproduction.

Reproductive health includes family planning (including abortion), prevention of maternal mortality, promotion of child survival and development, and "safe" sex, including the control of sexually transmitted diseases (STDs).

Improving reproductive health requires access to information, choice of contraception, maternal and child health services, and the prevention and treatment of STDs. Three kinds of research can support these goals.

Technological research for ensuring improved contraception faces special impediments: liability and regulatory constraints hinder product development, as do shifts in the political climate regarding reproductive rights. In 1970 there were 13 major pharmaceutical companies conducting research and development on new contraceptives, nine of which were in the United States. By 1987 this number had dwindled to four such companies, with only one in the United States.

A priority list of new or improved contraceptive methods that would benefit those of different income levels, gender, personal positions on abortion, and diverse life circumstances, includes:

- a new spermicide with antiviral properties
- a "once-a-month" pill effective as a menses-inducer
- a reliable ovulation predictor
- an improved oral contraceptive for women
- an improved intrauterine device
- an improved injectable contraceptive
- an easy, reliable, and reversible method of male sterilization
- an antifertility vaccine

Policy and socio-behavioral research is critical because the effectiveness of any technology is shaped as much by the user as by the technology itself. Policy research can help shape legislation and public attitudes toward accessible and high-quality services for all. Studying reproductive behavior can provide information on how and why individuals choose different contraceptive methods; what economic, social, and risk factors determine use; how the attitudes and behaviors of service providers influence choice and use of methods; and how cultural values and beliefs affect contraceptive selection and continuation.

Health systems research is essential to ensure a consistent, timely, and affordable supply of contraceptives to consumers. Where health care services are limited, health systems research to develop innovative coverage and follow-up procedures is especially critical.

Box 4.3 Deficiency of vitamin A: the quiet killer

Vitamin A, iron, and other micronutrients are essential for biological function. Their deficiency frequently results in severe health problems—such as blindness due to severe vitamin A deficiency or anemia due to iron deficiency. What appears to have been inadequately appreciated is the actual or potential impact of micronutrient deficiencies on other health problems. One example is endemic vitamin A deficiency, which is believed to be a significant yet quiet and indirect killer of children.

Recent field research among preschool-age children in Indonesia found a major indirect impact of vitamin A deficiency on childhood mortality. Preschool children with mild xerophthalmia (night blindness and/or Bitot's spots caused by vitamin A deficiency) experienced a mortality rate 4 to 12 times that of normal children. At least 16 percent of all deaths among children were directly associated with mild vitamin A deficiency. Follow-up intervention studies supplying vitamin A supplementation to randomly selected villages found that child survival in supplemented villages was about one-third higher than among children in villages receiving placebo supplementation.

If these findings are confirmed, the strategic implications would be astounding—up to one-third reduction of child mortality in vitamin A-deficient populations through supplementation. Because such findings hold enormous significance in shaping priorities for child survival interventions, hypotheses regarding this relationship require testing and confirmation from other settings. One hypothesis is that vitamin A deficiency causes broad systemic effects in the body, among them a reduced ability to resist infection, compromised epithelial cell functions in the gastrointestinal and respiratory tracts, and the increased risk of bacterial colonization in vulnerable organ systems.

Epidemiological and intervention research is currently underway in India, the Philippines, the Sudan, and other sites to validate the effect of supplementation with vitamin A on childhood survival among diverse populations. Preliminary findings from the India study suggest that the earlier Indonesian findings are relevant to another setting. Should these findings be confirmed in other sites, research will have identified an extremely important intervention for child survival.

Box 4.4 Applied research on essential drugs

The performance of health services everywhere critically depends on the availability and use of pharmaceutical products. Health workers cannot effectively treat many patients without drugs and vaccines. Indeed, public confidence in health workers and satisfaction with health services depend upon the maintenance of a reliable and affordable supply of drugs. Many countries spend one-third or more of health funds on drugs, much of it wasted because of unsafe and improper drug dispensing, prescription, and use, and because bacterial resistance often renders drugs ineffective. Indeed there are few factors that affect the cost-effectiveness of health services more than fostering the appropriate use and controlling and reducing the misuse of drugs.

Since Alma-Ata and the leadership of the WHO-led essential drug program, the use and supply of essential drugs has improved in many developing countries. Over 100 countries have developed lists of essential drugs; procurement and distribution systems have gradually improved; essential-drug training programs have been developed; and access to drugs has increased. The primary emphasis is on improving supply and ensuring that drugs are available and affordable in rough proportion to prevailing illness patterns.

Very little is known, however, about how providers make decisions about which drugs to prescribe and about how and why patients use—or don't use—medications. Behavioral research is urgently needed to improve the way pharmaceuticals are prescribed, dispensed, and used. Such research would:

- evaluate the impact of current pharmaceutical policies on drug use patterns;
- define the economic and clinical scope of particular drug use problems;
- delineate the motivations and incentives among providers and consumers for misuse of pharmaceuticals;
- determine the most efficient and cost-effective regulatory, managerial, and educational interventions for promoting effective drug use.

Research along these lines has begun in a variety of countries, including Sri Lanka, Zimbabwe, Nepal, and Tanzania. In addition, an International Network for the Rational Use of Drugs (INRUD) has recently been formed with support from WHO, the Pew Charitable Trusts, and the Swedish International Development Agency. INRUD is a cooperative arrangement among clinical researchers, behavioral scientists, health professionals, policymakers, and health managers in selected developing countries to improve the clinical impact and cost-effectiveness of pharmaceuticals. Composed of country core groups supported by a central unit, the network will serve as a vehicle for development of regional and national capacities to design and implement research and action.

been little research attention to coping with the growing problems of drug, alcohol, and tobacco addiction.

Setting Research Priorities

The priorities for health research should be strongly influenced by the anticipated health impact of the interventions expected to result from the research. Although quantitative methods are available to assess health impact, all priority-setting exercises are shaped by assumptions which can significantly influence the outcome. How is health defined and measured? How are health problems classified and grouped? What criteria are used? Who sets priorities for whom?

Most action-oriented priority-setting methods are based upon cost-effectiveness measures of health impact per unit expenditure. Table 4.5 (page 44) shows the results of one method of assessing the relative importance of different health problems in Ghana. The problems were ranked according to their significance as determined by the number of years of potential life lost due to specific diseases.[4] To complete a priority-setting analysis, it would be necessary also to estimate the costs of addressing various problems. The results would provide a framework to assist in the allocation of resources to address the diseases responsible for the most years of potential life lost.

No method of setting priorities can rest solely on numerical estimates. The recent debate over "selective primary health care" revolved as much around a set of political, social, and ethical issues as around technical differences[5]. Priority-setting cannot help but reflect ethical judgments regarding the value of human life and the best way of conserving or enhancing it.

In addition to problem significance and cost of intervention, a research agenda should be influenced by factors that favor successful execution—scientific feasibility, intellectual challenge, and the human and organizational capability of the research community. Other key issues in shaping research priorities are who sets priorities for whom and the time horizon of research benefits.

Who sets priorities for whom?

Priorities are determined at many levels of population: the family, the community, and the national, regional, and international levels. These are not necessarily in agreement; the needs expressed by a community may differ from the priorities determined by a national policymaker. Participatory research is an approach designed to involve the intended beneficiaries, for example the community, in setting priorities and conducting the research. Country-level priority setting should take

into account variations in needs among subnational units. International research priorities should reflect national priorities weighted, for example, to help countries with the greatest health needs and the fewest resources. Any process designed to set priorities, therefore, should not lose sight of the fundamental questions: whose voic-

---

Box 4.5 Behavioral health in developing countries

Behavioral health problems span a range of psychosocial conditions that as a group are inadequately recognized in most developing countries. Severe psychiatric disease, for example, affects at least 2 percent of those living in developing countries, and the lifetime probability of major mental illness is about 10 percent. At any given time, 5 to 10 percent of the population suffers from anxiety, depressive disorders, and other psychosocial problems seriously affecting daily functioning. Although the diagnosis is often missed, up to 20 percent of the patients attending primary care clinics meet accepted criteria for depression or panic disorder. Epilepsy affects up to 5 percent of the people in the developing world, several times the rate in industrialized countries. Up to 10 percent of the world's children and adolescents suffer from behavior disorders. Smoking, alcohol use, and illicit drug use are all on the rise in societies undergoing rapid developmental change. Substance abuse contributes significantly to tragically high rates of violence, spouse and child abuse, child abandonment, suicide, and accidents.

Effective treatments are now at hand for many of these conditions. In an experimental field study supported by WHO, over 90 percent of patients with selected major psychiatric illnesses were successfully treated with medications from a limited pharmacopoeia. Primary care givers can be trained in as little as five hours to reliably diagnose major mental illnesses. Up to 60 percent of the individuals with epilepsy in the developing world could be treated effectively with anti-convulsants at an annual cost of less than $0.05 per person in the population covered, or $10.00 per case.

Behavioral health must be given higher priority among national governments and the international funding community. A primary aim should be the development of a cadre of competent researchers in developing countries themselves. Research is needed on how to train primary care providers in the recognition and treatment of the common major psychiatric conditions. Children, women in their childbearing years, and young adolescents are prime candidates for prevention strategies. Similarly, strategies for case finding and treatment of epilepsy are needed. Other concerns, such as the epidemiology of drug and alcohol abuse in developing societies, require a solid data base. All such research should incorporate ethnographic awareness to ensure that the questions being asked, and the data sought, are appropriate to the cultural and social setting.

Table 4.5 Ranking of health problems in Ghana by years of potential life lost, 1981

RANK	DISEASE	PERCENTAGE OF YEARS OF POTENTIAL LIFE LOST
1	Malaria	10.2
2	Measles	7.3
3	Pneumonia	5.8
4	Sickle cell disease	5.5
5	Malnutrition	5.5
6	Prematurity	5.2
7	Birth injury	5.2
8	Accidents	4.7
9	Gastroenteritis	4.5

Source: Ghana Health Assessment Project Team 1981

es are heard, whose views prevail and, thus, whose health interests are advanced.

Time horizon of benefits

One challenge in setting a research agenda is the trade-off between meeting current health needs and generating future health benefits. The research that guides and supports most health policy and management decisions has a near-term horizon. Such research should be relevant and communicated in a usable form to policymakers and those involved in action. Longer time horizons are needed, however, to realize large future benefits from advances in basic knowledge and the development of new technologies. Longer time horizon research groups should be insulated from demands for immediate operational advice and more able to pursue an intellectually driven research agenda in a stable and supportive environment. Every country would be well served by a balance of both types of research, although the relative mix will vary depending on the country's stage of development.

Conclusions

1. The major causes of death in developing countries are the infectious and parasitic diseases, and reproductive and perinatal health problems. Chronic and degenerative diseases, such as cancer and circulatory diseases, are of growing importance. Many developing countries are already facing the double burden of pre- and post-transitional health problems simultaneously.

2. Health problems show great diversity among developing countries, among regions within countries, and among communities. Each country should make internal decisions regarding its particular mix of research, given its own health problems and its own stage of development. Country-specific research, critical to all countries at all stages of development, is needed to promote national independence, choice, and capacity in setting health priorities.

3. Setting global research priorities is a worldwide challenge involving the combined efforts of many nations. Priority setting at the international level is important if the relatively neglected health problems of developing countries are to receive the attention they deserve in the interest of global health equity. Global priorities should be built upon an upward synthesis of national priorities, rather than imposed from the top down.

4. Some high-priority health problems, such as tropical diseases, human reproduction, and AIDS, are receiving international research funding. Many other important problems appear to be comparatively neglected, such as acute respiratory infections, tuberculosis, sexually transmitted diseases, and injury. Moreover, diseases that cause morbidity rather than mortality appear to be comparatively neglected, such as behavioral health problems, skin diseases, and diseases that cause blindness and other serious disabilities that interfere with independent living.

5. Problems that are not classified by disease also require research attention, such as the financing of health services, the development of health information systems, and the waste and misuse of therapeutic drugs.

CHAPTER 5

Research in Developing Countries

*T*his chapter presents our findings on the state of health research in developing countries. Our assessment rests on our own first-hand experience, on extensive consultations with developing-country scientists and health leaders, on documentary evidence, and on special papers written at our request.

Research Output

Because of the enormous diversity of developing countries and the limited availability of organized information on health research, we sponsored special surveys in 10 selected countries.[1] Country selection was not random; rather, it was contingent upon the identification of colleagues in developing countries who were prepared to undertake systematic review of health research activities in their countries. Table 5.1 shows that while the case-study countries are not representative of the entire developing world, they illustrate a wide range of development circumstances as indicated by per capita GNP, population size, geographic location, and other development measures.

The surveys were, in nearly every case, first attempts in those countries to gather systematic information on health research. The results have many imperfections, and the data from different countries are not strictly comparable. Nevertheless, they provide insight into the range and depth of health research in developing countries. While the situation varies from country to country, in the developing world as a whole there is significant capacity for health research, with substantial numbers of scientists in many institutions working on research projects (Box 5.1). Their dedication and energy are impressive, but the quality of their work is hampered by severe constraints. The individual case studies revealed a compendium of common constraints to research related to professional development, the work environment, and the macro-environment (Figure 5.1).

The country case studies also yielded information on the pattern of research investments in developing countries (Figure 5.2). The data from Thailand, the Philippines, and Mexico show, not surprisingly, a heavy dominance by clinical, biomedical, and laboratory research, ranging from 60 to 90 percent of total health research expenditures. Research activity was small on health information systems,

> *The clearer the voices of our researchers, the better would politicians hear. . . . But even more important is that we realize that our own understanding of our countries is a fundamental requirement for balanced international policy debate.*
>
> **Alfredo R. A. Bengzon**
> *Secretary of Health, The Philippines*

Table 5.1 Case-study countries: selected indicators, 1986

COUNTRY 1[a]	PER CAPITA GNP (DOLLARS) 2	POPULATION (MILLIONS) 3	CRUDE BIRTH RATE PER 1,000 POPULATION 4	LIFE EXPECTANCY AT BIRTH (YEARS) 5	INFANT MORTALITY PER 1,000 LIVE BIRTHS 6	PERCENTAGE OF AGE GROUP EN- ROLLED IN PRIMARY EDUCATION: MALE 7[b]	FEMALE 8[b]
Ethiopia	120	43.5	47	46	155	44	28
Bangladesh	160	103.2	41	50	121	70	50
Mali	180	7.6	48	47	144	29	17
India	290	781.4	32	57	86	107	76
Philippines	560	57.3	35	63	46	105	106
Zimbabwe	620	8.7	45	58	74	135	128
Egypt	760	49.7	34	61	88	94	76
Thiland	810	52.6	25	64	41	—	—
Brazil	1,810	138.4	29	65	65	108	99
Mexico	1,860	80.2	29	68	48	116	114

[a] Listed according to per capita GNP.

[b] Estimated ratio of pupils of all ages in primary school to the population of primary-school-age children, 1985. In several cases the total enrollment is larger than the number of children of primary-school age.

Source: World Bank 1988

field epidemiology, demography, behavioral sciences, economics, and management. While these data do not translate automatically into the two categories of country-specific and global research, they suggest that country-specific research has been relatively neglected in most developing countries. This impression was reinforced at Commission workshops held in 1989 in Dhaka, Harare, Rio de Janeiro, and Cairo, and in 1990 in Puebla, Mexico. In all cases, local health researchers coming

from all disciplines agreed that country-specific research has been seriously neglected and requires special attention.

Another source of information about health research in developing countries is the record of publications. The Excerpta Medica bibliographical data base for 1988 showed 16,220 publications (or 5.6 percent of the 286,095 publications from all areas) whose first authors lived in developing countries. These data have well-

---

Box 5.1 Research capacity in case-study countries

Case-study data show substantial diversity among developing countries and a considerable number of professionally trained health researchers in some countries. As would be expected, the number of researchers per million population rises as per capita GNP rises. In some cases, notably Ethiopia and Bangladesh, a significant number of expatriate researchers is included.

Country	Health researchers	Health researchers per million population
Ethiopia	300	6.9
Bangladesh	150	1.5
Mali	10	1.3
Philippines	939	16.4
Zimbabwe	125	14.4
Brazil	8,521	61.6
Mexico	4,380	54.6

Source: Commission country studies

The case studies also noted that there are numerous institutions conducting health research in developing countries. The pattern of institutional research activity differs among countries. In the Philippines, for example, the bulk of the health research is conducted in roughly equal shares by private and public universities; only 12.5 percent is carried out by governmental agencies. In Mexico nearly the opposite is true: 75 percent of health research projects are carried out in governmental institutions. In Zimbabwe a single university, the University of Zimbabwe, carries out about 80 percent of all research projects.

Although we did not request data on numbers of health research projects, the studies from the Philippines, Zimbabwe, and Thailand reported that in each case several hundred projects were underway.

known weaknesses: they include publications by expatriates; they omit many local publications; and they are biased toward publications in English. Nevertheless, they support the conclusion from our country studies that there is an active health research community in developing countries—small by the standards of industrialized countries, but productive in spite of many handicaps.

Researchers

Well-compensated, professionally secure, full-time researchers with the freedom to determine their own research agenda are exceedingly uncommon in developing countries. Researchers typically face limited career paths, few opportunities for promotion, intellectual isolation, and restricted choice of research agenda. Low salaries, especially in comparison to the financial rewards of private clinical practice, work in industry, or administration, discourage promising young researchers. There are often pressures to take on additional income-generating activities that divert time and attention from research. These constraints to professional development compromise research productivity and limit the appeal that research careers hold for bright young professionals.

Institutions

Health research is undertaken in governmental departments, free-standing research institutes or centers, universities and medical schools, and nongovernmental agencies.

Some developing-country institutions rank among world leaders in health research, but these are rare. In most developing countries the tradition of modern scientific research is young, and the institutional infrastructure is fragile. Resource constraints—inadequate facilities, lack of technicians and support staff, unreliable equipment and vital supplies, and unstable budgetary support —compromise many aspects of research. There is often limited access to information and research journals. The concept of peer review and constructive criticism has yet to penetrate deeply into the research practices of many developing countries.[2] As a

consequence, research quality, admittedly a difficult parameter to measure, tends to be marginal, limiting confidence in the usefulness of research results.

The environment for research

Most of the scientific and institutional failings are conditioned by economic and political forces in the broader environment. Perhaps most significant is the lack of demand for or social appreciation of research. Public awareness of the utility of research is low, and research demand among politicians and policymakers is weak in the face of budgetary pressures and competing priorities.

In many instances the research process is not adequately matched with the needs of the beneficiaries or policymakers. In some cases, scientists may neglect im-

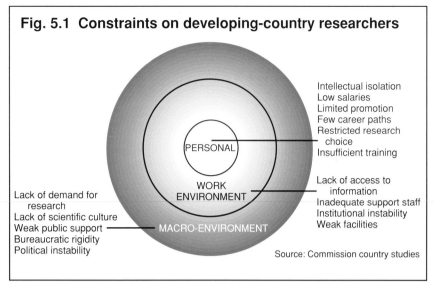

Fig. 5.1 Constraints on developing-country researchers

PERSONAL

WORK ENVIRONMENT

MACRO-ENVIRONMENT

Intellectual isolation
Low salaries
Limited promotion
Few career paths
Restricted research choice
Insufficient training

Lack of access to information
Inadequate support staff
Institutional instability
Weak facilities

Lack of demand for research
Lack of scientific culture
Weak public support
Bureaucratic rigidity
Political instability

Source: Commission country studies

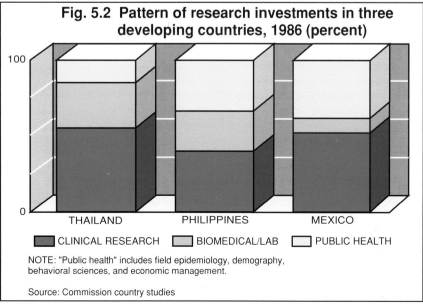

Fig. 5.2 Pattern of research investments in three developing countries, 1986 (percent)

THAILAND   PHILIPPINES   MEXICO

■ CLINICAL RESEARCH   ▨ BIOMEDICAL/LAB   □ PUBLIC HEALTH

NOTE: "Public health" includes field epidemiology, demography, behavioral sciences, and economic management.

Source: Commission country studies

portant local opportunities in favor of emulating the models and subject priorities of the scientific establishment in industrialized countries. Other serious constraints on research are inconsistent policies and bureaucratic rigidity. The management of high-quality research requires not only institutional stability, but also more flexible procedures than those that are used in the management of public bureaucracies.

Most important, the economic situation in many developing countries has led to budgetary cutbacks which are undermining the morale of researchers and the stability of research institutions. In many countries, research salaries in real terms have fallen dramatically. Urgent remedial actions are needed to curb large-scale emigration of the best scientists to more secure situations in international agencies and industrialized countries. The situation is further complicated by the needs of research establishments in industrialized countries to attract bright students from abroad in order to compensate for a smaller cohort of domestic students interested in scientific careers. To avoid the loss of critical human resources, some developing countries, such as Mexico, have instituted innovative programs to retain and support key national scientists (Box 5.2).

Another concern is the degree of dependence on foreign funding for research activities in developing countries (Figure 5.3). Even in cases in which domestic resources support half or more of total research expenditures, local funds may be so heavily committed to salaries and maintenance of facilities as to leave little flexibility to support direct research costs.

Foreign funding of research, usually in the form of project support, can have both positive and negative effects. Deleterious consequences include the short duration of funding, the "artificial growth and fragmentation" of research programs and institutions, and the imposition of a foreign research agenda on national priorities.[3] If foreign funders do not help to build indigenous research capacity, their externally imposed research priorities may overwhelm an already stretched pool of researchers, dissipating their focus and productivity. Much longer duration of support by foreign funders is necessary to build national research capability. Much stronger national research plans and domestic priorities need to be established within developing countries so that foreign research investments can be rationalized and made more effective.

Research Dissemination and Use

Research can be undertaken within specialized research institutions or as a component of an action agency (governmental or nongovernmental). Either arrangement has both advantages and weaknesses. Full-time research bodies can focus attention on a long-term research agenda, but they may undertake their work in relative isolation from policy and action. Action agencies are more likely to formulate critically relevant questions and have inherently strong motivation to utilize research results, but they tend to limit their focus to short-

---

Box 5.2 Mexico: a special program for national research

Mexico's National Researchers System (SNI) is a publicly supported yet entirely independent system to retain and support outstanding Mexican scientists working in the country. The aims of the SNI are to strengthen the capacity of Mexican researchers and to increase the quality of Mexican research. Created in 1984, the SNI was launched as an expression of presidential commitment to research-based development.

A group of distinguished Mexican scientists was asked to propose a national mechanism that could effectively sustain research in a country faced with a severe economic crisis. They proposed a system based on peer review that would function independent of political or collegial pressure. The assessment of scientists is conducted exclusively by researchers, and the SNI functions as an accreditation system for researchers assigned to one of three levels. Researchers at the higher levels evaluate those at the lower levels; researchers at the highest level review their peers.

The SNI has picked out not only the best researchers in Mexico today, but also the young researchers and postgraduates who will constitute Mexico's scientific community of tomorrow. SNI-selected researchers receive a tax-free salary supplement that may represent over half their total income, and these supplements are indexed to inflation. The SNI imposes no requirements on researchers other than periodic peer review and full-time commitment to research.

The total extra cost of SNI represents a negligible fraction of Mexico's research and education expenditure. The program has had a noticeable impact on scientific production. As can be seen in the table below, the average number of publications per researcher increased markedly for the three levels (plus candidates for entry) of medical researchers after the SNI was launched.

Category of Researcher	Publications per researcher	
	Before SNI	**After SNI**
	1982-84	1984-87
Candidate	1.0	7.0
Level I	7.0	8.7
Level II	9.7	10.8
Level III (highest)	16.5	24.3

term research, and the research work is often interrupted by other demands on the researcher's time.

As a general rule, country-specific research should be closely linked to action. Dissemination and use of such research require strong linkages with consumers, policymakers, and the community. Global research should also be linked to those who will use the results, but long-term advances may require greater independence and autonomy from the pressing needs of action. In comparison with industry, which shapes its research agenda to marketing signals and invests proportionately more funds in dissemination, health research systems have paid far too little attention to mechanisms for the dissemination and use of research results. Much stronger efforts are needed to ensure that consumers of research participate in the formulation of research activities and that research results are disseminated to appropriate audiences. Some countries have recognized these gaps and are undertaking innovative actions to address them (Box 5.3).

Education and Science

A broad-based scientific culture, beginning with basic literacy, is an underlying requirement for effective

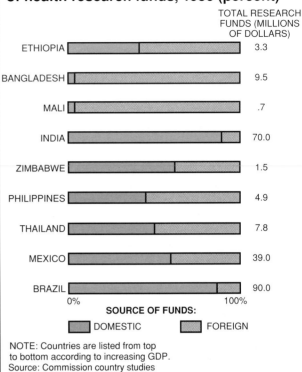

Fig. 5.3 Domestic and foreign sources of health research funds, 1986 (percent)

TOTAL RESEARCH FUNDS (MILLIONS OF DOLLARS)

ETHIOPIA	3.3
BANGLADESH	9.5
MALI	.7
INDIA	70.0
ZIMBABWE	1.5
PHILIPPINES	4.9
THAILAND	7.8
MEXICO	39.0
BRAZIL	90.0

0%   SOURCE OF FUNDS: 100%

DOMESTIC   FOREIGN

NOTE: Countries are listed from top to bottom according to increasing GDP.
Source: Commission country studies

Box 5.3 Linking researchers and policymakers in the Philippines

The Philippine Institute of Development Studies (PIDS) is a government research institution engaged in long-term policy-oriented research. Its mandate is to develop a research program that will provide the government with an informational and analytical basis for its planning and policy work. Supported by a recent grant from the International Health Policy Program (IHPP), PIDS has undertaken six studies relevant to the Philippines' health sector. PIDS' methods of linking the research and policy communities through shared research priority setting and regular mechanisms for research dissemination are noteworthy and potentially useful to other countries, including:

Setting the research agenda In 1986 PIDS conducted a two-day health policy workshop to identify country-specific priority issues in health in the Philippines. The workshop, attended by research analysts, government health leaders, and private practitioners, featured reviews about the Philippine health system, four of which were published. Reviews were also synthesized to form the basis for a research agenda, from which the six IHPP-funded studies were chosen.

Research management The six IHPP research projects are contracted to five institutions forming a consortium under PIDS supervision. A steering committee consists of two high-level government policy advisors, in addition to four research advisors, research analysts, and the PIDS research director. The committee meets regularly to discuss research problems and to provide direction. Draft research

reports are circulated as PIDS working papers for peer evaluation and are reviewed by the steering committee.

Research utilization and advocacy The involvement of the Department of Health in the critical stages of the research process—agenda preparation, steering committee meetings, dissemination of findings—helps to ensure that research findings are both useful and used. A memorandum of agreement between the department and PIDS specifies each agency's role in the research process; this is necessary because the government is both the primary user of research and the primary source of data.

In addition to these formal mechanisms, many informal channels encourage linkages between researchers and policymakers. PIDS staff have been invited to congressional hearings to comment on health sector issues; other users of health research have access to PIDS studies and journals. Research activities from other institutions are made known to PIDS research analysts through a PIDS information clearinghouse project.

PIDS is expanding the health research agenda and making policy analysis a permanent feature of its health research program. It is establishing contacts with donors to solicit support for health research, and is planning with the Department of Health to become the primary health policy research base in the country. An important result of its work is that the momentum generated by PIDS so far has attracted a number of young research analysts to the health field, enhancing health research capacity in the Philippines.

Box 5.4 Shaping medical education to country-specific health needs

In the 1970s a number of universities around the world embarked on an innovative plan to provide health professionals with skills and orientations more closely attuned to the health needs of their communities. In 1979, with the support of PAHO and WHO, they formed the **Network of Community-Oriented Educational Institutions for Health Sciences** and established a secretariat at the University of Limburg in the Netherlands. The network has grown to include more than 100 medical faculties and health science institutions, of which 45 are full members. Over half of all member institutions are from developing countries.

Network task forces and project groups focus on community-based education, innovation in curriculum planning, faculty and institutional development, and the university role in intersectoral linkages. Mutual institutional support is fostered through communications, consultations, and exchanges. At the September 1989 biennial meeting, about 300 participants discussed the interaction between universities and health systems in national health development. A new initiative, the University Partnership Project, will help a selected number of institutions involve students in health systems research as an integral part of their education. This will be done within a research program that is collaboratively designed by the university, community representatives, and appropriate government agencies.

Sharing a similar concern for more relevant medical education, the **World Federation for Medical Education**, consisting of regional medical education associations, has organized discussions aimed at enhancing the relevance of medical education. Led by a planning commission assembled in 1984, federation events culminated in a 1988 world conference held in Edinburgh. A preparatory document was reviewed at national and regional meetings, leading to recommendations that were placed before the world conference. An Edinburgh Declaration urged the world's medical educators and others to consider specific actions aimed at overcoming the dichotomy between the direction of medical schools and the health needs of countries. The declaration called for ". . . action, vigorous leadership and political will to alter the character of medical education so that it meets the needs of the societies in which it is situated." Subsequently, a series of ministerial consultations, initially in Europe and Africa, has brought together ministers of health and education, along with regional leaders in medical education. Specific national and regional projects are now in the planning stage.

research generation, demand, and use. Also important is the quality of basic science education and university and graduate education.

Medical education is critically important because physicians dominate the health sector. In many developing countries, medical education is not meeting national health needs. Problems such as irrelevant curricula, over-production of physicians, geographic maldistribution, domination by private clinical practice, and lack

of research and population-based instruction are generating severe problems for the health sector. A few innovative actions for improving the quality and relevance of medical education and research are underway in both developing and industrialized countries. Two examples are described in Box 5.4.

To promote and support research, many countries have established national research councils or academies. These, in turn, may be linked to regional or

Box 5.5 The Third World Academy of Sciences

Weak public recognition and political support, intellectual isolation, and insufficient peer support faced by scientists in developing countries are being tackled by a new organization established to honor excellence in the work of Third World researchers and to nurture the development of young scientists. Launched in 1985 on the initiative of Professor Abdus Salam, a Nobel Prize-winning physicist from Pakistan, the Third World Academy of Sciences is an international forum to unite distinguished men and women of science from developing countries.

The academy's membership as of late 1989 consisted of 198 elected members representing 47 developing countries. In addition to directly encouraging scientists, the academy also works to improve research conditions, to promote contact and exchange, to raise public awareness, and to support research on key problems of developing countries.

In a recent speech, Dr. Salam observed that "the profession of science and science-based technology is hardly a respectable—hardly a valid—profession in the South." He noted that industrialized countries spend 2.0 to 2.5 percent of GNP on science and technology compared to less than 0.3 percent spent by most developing countries. On average, industrialized countries are spending nine times more, as a share of GNP, on science and technology than are Third World countries. Dr. Salam urges upon Third World leaders a national investment of at least 2 percent of GNP for indigenous science and technology development which would support immediate and sustained build-up and utilization of the neglected community of Third World scientists: "Their numbers need to be multiplied so that they constitute a critical size; they have to be given proper recognition, provided with scientific literature and infrastructure, international contacts and provisions for their work, and guaranteed tolerance for their beliefs. . . . With careful nurturing and proper trust, they surely have the capability of transforming the South."

international councils and academies. The Third World Academy of Sciences is an example of an international body promoting science in developing countries (Box 5.5). Although young, these national and international councils and academies can perform useful functions by according recognition to high-quality research and by generating broader support.

Conclusions

1. Research on health in most developing countries suffers serious constraints, including limited opportunities for career advancement and professional development, weak and unstable institutional environments, and insufficient and erratic funding. The lack of appreciation of the importance of research has resulted in low social esteem and poor salary structures for scientists.

2. In spite of the constraints, there exists an active health research community in many parts of the developing world that is often unrecognized. Strong and sustained efforts to overcome constraints could result in steady increases in research capacity in developing countries and possibly attract back some of the developing-country scientists who are making international contributions from bases in industrialized countries.

3. Research capacity in the fields most relevant to country-specific research, including epidemiology, social/policy sciences, and management, is seriously neglected in most developing countries, as is also the case in most industrialized countries.

4. The training of personnel for health services and health research is often inappropriate to the health needs of developing countries. Curricular reform and strengthening of medical education are needed to redirect the training of health professionals to meet the health needs of their own communities.

5. In many developing countries, domestic research funds are tied up in infrastructure and salaries. Foreign funds, therefore, often disproportionately dictate the research agenda. Stronger national research plans and priorities are urgently needed so that foreign funds can be more effectively used.

6. The linkage between research and the utilization of research results needs to be strengthened by more participation of research users in setting the objectives and timetable for research projects and by communicating the results more effectively to potential users.

CHAPTER 6

Research in Industrialized Countries and International Centers

This chapter examines two subjects: first, the involvement of industrialized-country institutions in research on the health problems of developing countries, and second, the value of international health research centers for addressing developing-country health problems. Lastly, because the agricultural sector has a pattern of autonomous international research centers that many view as successful, the chapter discusses the extent to which the agricultural model may be applicable to the health sector.

Industrialized-Country Research

Industrialized-country scientists and institutions are overwhelmingly focused on the development of technologies for the diseases of more affluent societies. Nevertheless, a small share of their efforts is directed toward health problems of developing countries. This small share, as noted in Chapter 3, is large in relation to developing-country research expenditures, so that at present about half the research funds directed at health problems of developing nations are expended in industrialized countries. Furthermore, researchers in industrialized countries, because they work in a favorable scientific environment, often are able to contribute disproportionately to scientific advances.

The power of modern health research is currently being demonstrated and tested in the case of AIDS. While much remains to be done, the progress in AIDS research thus far has been remarkable: within five years of the first clear identification of the disease, the viruses had been identified, specific diagnostic tests had been developed for general application, and the basic epidemiology of disease transmission had been discovered. Looking ahead, large contributions can be anticipated from researchers in industrialized countries not only on AIDS but on many other health problems of developing countries, ranging from particular diseases to broad issues like nutrition and population growth.

A historically important role has been played by free-standing and university-based research institutions in Europe and North America in addressing the health problems of developing countries.[1] Foremost among their contributions is advanced research in biomedicine and public health. Advanced training is also provided to developing-country as well as industrialized-country professionals. Technical assistance, information, and direct services are other valuable activities.

> *The truth is that medicine, professedly founded on observation, is as sensitive to outside influences, political, religious, philosophical, imaginative, as is the barometer to the changes of atmospheric density. [There is] a closer relation between the Medical Sciences and the conditions of Society and the general thought of the time than would at first be suspected.*
>
> **Oliver Wendell Holmes**
> *Nineteenth-century American physician and author*

Box 6.1 The future role of European tropical institutes

European tropical institutes have a long tradition of research and program involvement mainly with African countries. With changing contexts, especially the unification of Europe in 1992, major rethinking of the future role of these institutions is underway.

Some people are pessimistic over the future role of the tropical institutes. Many faculty have only short-term funding available, which creates career insecurity. A further area of concern is the relative isolation of the institutes from the research community of their home country because they concentrate on "exotic diseases." This is a counterproductive attitude at a time when a comprehensive approach to problems is needed.

A more realistic and optimistic view is that these institutions are important assets with strong prospects for the future. Their roles are now being redefined in four crucial areas:

1. Because of their longstanding involvement, the tropical institutes provide a wealth of experience and are valuable places for researchers from developing countries to take courses, spend time in research, and meet and share experiences with colleagues.

2. The institutes are multi-disciplinary, carrying out a broad range of types of research from biomedical to socio-epidemiological. This mix needs to be maintained. The institutes also provide important quality control functions for research results from around the world.

3. The tropical institutes support diversity and independence in the choice of research topics, which is extremely important in the face of the tendency for research to be driven by specific agendas dictated by funding agencies.

4. The institutes are strong bases for exchanges and for research collaboration with developing countries. While interactive centers within developing countries should be generated and managed not by foreign but by local scientists, continuity of cooperation between scientists of developed and developing countries is a necessary and mutually enriching process.

Western European research institutes continue to evolve rapidly, and they may well undergo further transformation after the union of Europe in 1992 (Box 6.1). The older institutions often focus on the tropical diseases, with the London School of Hygiene and Tropical Medicine and the Royal Tropical Institute in Amsterdam perhaps the best known.[2] Newer groups have emerged in the past several decades, broadening into the social

Box 6.2 Japan's international cooperation in health

Paralleling its astounding economic growth, Japan is rapidly overtaking the United States as the largest source of foreign aid. Japan's development assistance policies have progressed through a series of stages, and the country is now assuming greater global responsibilities. Japan's proposed foreign aid budget for 1989 exceeded the U.S. allocation for 1988 by more than $1 billion. This budget marks the first step of Prime Minister Noboru Takeshita's June 1988 promise to double Japan's official development assistance over five years—from $25 billion in 1983-87, to at least $50 billion in 1988-92—and to improve such assistance through increasing the share of grants and untied aid.

At the same time, major changes are underway in Japanese institutions involved in international cooperation in health. The Japan International Cooperation Agency (JICA) is planning to balance its system for providing assistance between a "request basis" and an "offer basis." The Ministry of Health and Welfare has established a Department of International Medical Cooperation at the National Medical Center Hospital of Tokyo, and also has created an Office of International Cooperation, separate from the Division of International Affairs. In order to assist in these activities, the establishment of two foundations is in progress. The first, called the Foundation for International Medical Research, promotes health and medical research for development, and the second, the Foundation for Development of International Health, aims at strengthening the preventive component of Japan's health programs in the Third World. The Minister of Foreign Affairs, Taro Nakayama, who is a physician, emphasizes the need for health cooperation in Japan's foreign policy. Survey missions have already been sent to several nations involving the joint efforts of the ministries of health and welfare, education, and foreign affairs.

In the nongovernmental sector, Japan's Research Institute on Tuberculosis has long provided educational courses in English, supported by JICA, for researchers and practitioners from the developing world. As one of the few remaining major research institutes on tuberculosis in the world, Japan's facility seeks to fulfill a global responsibility in this field. Several Japanese universities have international health research centers, including the International Medical Research Center of Kobe University and the Institute of Tropical Medicine of Nagasaki University. And the University of Tokyo is now planning to begin a graduate level course about international health. During the course of the Commission's activities, commissioner Saburo Okita formed a special committee of distinguished Japanese scientists and leaders to advise him on matters related to the Commission's work.

These developments, along with the election of Dr. Hiroshi Nakajima as director-general of WHO, indicate that Japan will continue to expand its role in research for health and development and will continue to improve the quality of its international cooperation for health in developing countries.

sciences; some, such as the various institutes for development studies in Europe, have pursued health research within the context of socioeconomic development. The work of British nutrition institutes and French demography is well recognized internationally. Several important centers have been established in Scandinavia, and significant work is being undertaken by French scientists at the Pasteur Institutes in France and around the world.

In North America there are over two dozen schools of public health, and some medical schools, that undertake overseas work in health research. The oldest and largest is the Johns Hopkins School of Hygiene and Public Health. North America also has a half dozen leading nutrition research centers and nearly two dozen population research institutions, mostly based in universities. These educational institutions are joined by the recent growth of private professional firms that undertake contractual work from governmental agencies. Within the United States government, the most notable institutions are the National Institute of Allergy and Infectious Disease (NIAID) of the National Institutes of Health (NIH), and the Centers for Disease Control (CDC).

In Japan, institutional resources are just beginning to emerge in response to the country's rapidly expanding development assistance role. In preparation for Japan's growing international responsibilities, new programs and centers are being strengthened or established (Box 6.2).

Changing Roles

Industrialized-country researchers and institutions have crucial roles to play, especially in conducting leading-edge research and in helping to build research capacity in developing countries.

Because of their favorable research environments, institutions in industrialized countries can play major roles in capturing the extraordinary opportunities offered by advanced research techniques to find new diagnostics, vaccines, and therapeutic agents to deal with health problems in developing countries. Similar opportunities exist in the social sciences—especially in improving methodologies for their use in health research.

Significant gains in efficiency in conducting such research can be achieved through stronger collaboration between industrialized and developing countries, which puts industrialized-country researchers directly in touch with the reality of Third World problems.[3] Such collaboration has two-way benefits. There are mutually beneficial opportunities for collaborative research to address shared problems. This need is obvious with problems such as AIDS and other viral diseases (Box 6.3) and environmental health; indeed, some have argued that the field-testing of an effective AIDS vaccine and protection from environmental health threats are not possible without cooperation from developing countries. In addition, as industrialized countries cope with escalating costs and technological advances, they can learn from the lower-cost health models and innovations established in developing countries, which cannot afford the profligate practices of the industrialized world.[4]

Research collaboration between institutions in industrialized and in developing countries, if conducted with mutual respect and common objectives, can be a major means for building research capacity in both developing and industrialized countries. Moreover, research institutions in industrialized countries have a ma-

---

Box 6.3 Viral diseases: early recognition of shared health threats

The potential threat of devastating new viral diseases underlines the importance of international cooperation in epidemiological research to identify new patterns of disease and modes of transmission, and biological research to study the behavior of viruses and to develop tools for diagnosis, treatment, and prevention. The speed and extent of international movement of people can rapidly transform a local disease into a global epidemic.

AIDS has dramatized the difficulties of coping with a new disease. It is, however, but one of more than a dozen new or newly recognized viral diseases infecting humans that have been identified in recent decades. Others include a new form of hepatitis, several varieties of hemorrhagic fever (originating in Argentina, Bolivia, Zaire, Sudan, and Korea), Marburg disease (West Germany from a tropical virus in Ugandan monkey cells used for tissue culture), Rift Valley fever (Africa), Kyasanur Forest disease (India), O'Ny-ong-nyong (Uganda) and Rocio encephalitis (Brazil).

The source of newly recognized viral infections in humans is often not known, although some may have transferred from wild or domestic animals. As populations expand into wilderness areas and come in contact with infected animals, as ecological changes occur such as those resulting from the construction of the Aswan High Dam, or as living conditions deteriorate as the result of poverty, war, and intense urbanization, a virus that was often innocuous in the host animal may cause severe disease in the humans first infected.

Global disease surveillance and mobilization of scientific capability worldwide are important back-up resources to detect and deal with an epidemic. Research capability is needed in the first instance, however, in developing countries, where most of the new diseases initially appear. Since good local research capability cannot be created overnight, it is essential to build and sustain such capacity continually if new threats are to be promptly detected and effectively controlled.

Table 6.1 Total publicly funded health research in industrialized countries, 1986 (millions of dollars)

COUNTRY	TOTAL PUBLICLY FUNDED HEALTH RESEARCH		
	TOTAL EXPENDITURE 1	PERCENT OF GDP 2	PERCENT OF TOTAL HEALTH EXPENDITURE 3
Austria	174	.19	2.7
Australia	86	.05	0.7
Belgium	102	.09	1.4
Bulgaria	11	-	-
Canada	202	.06	0.7
Czechoslovakia	35	-	-
Denmark	106	.13	1.9
Finland	37	.05	0.8
France	807	.11	1.2
Germany, Fed. Rep.	1,329	.15	1.9
Germany, Dem. Rep.	44	-	-
Greece	12	.00	-
Hungary	19	.08	-
Ireland	4	.02	0.2
Israel	88	-	-
Italy	520	.09	1.4
Japan	1,920	.10	1.5
Netherlands	312	.18	2.1
New Zealand	17	.07	1.0
Norway	90	.13	1.9
Poland	38	-	-
Portugal	14	.06	1.0
Romania	7	-	-
Spain	32	.01	0.2
Sweden	288	.22	2.3
Switzerland	150	.11	1.4
United Kingdom	393	.07	1.2
United States	7,900	.19	1.8
Soviet Union	320	-	-
Yugoslavia	36	.06	-
TOTAL	**15,096**		

Source: Commission estimates

jor role to play in providing advanced training for researchers. As the numbers of scientists in developing countries grow, it will be particularly important for research institutions in developing countries to assume greater training responsibilities and for industrialized-country institutions to offer increased fellowship opportunities for those at advanced research levels and at mid-career in both the biological and social sciences. Through such experiences, the capacity of developing-country colleagues, increasingly nurtured by international collaboration, can be significantly enhanced. Forms of co-equal research and training exchanges between developed and developing-country institutions need to be facilitated.

In an interdependent world, compelling grounds exist to reinforce and extend appropriate patterns of relationships between industrialized and developing countries. Old and established patterns of interaction need to be assessed afresh and redefined where necessary. A culture of partnership, equality, and collaboration should be encouraged.

In order to respond to these opportunities, however, industrialized-country groups must overcome serious constraints. Limited, perhaps even declining, public funds have resulted in unstable financial support to industrialized-country researchers and institutions. This translates into unstable research programs, a lack of career opportunities for scientists, and an inability to attract talented young graduates to the field of health and development. In addition, field opportunities in developing countries, including technical or professional assistance roles, are no longer as numerous, welcomed, or clear-cut as they have been in the past.

The funding practices of donor groups have had important effects on the capability of some industrialized-country institutions. The pioneering work of some North American foundations on tropical disease research has been critical, for example, in nurturing and maintaining research contributions from both industrialized and developing-country groups (Box 6.4). On the other hand, contractual grant systems used in several major industrialized countries have forced many research groups to become technical contractors to donor agencies. While such practices may obtain relevant services for donor agencies, they are financially unstable and breed a competitive contract culture that can be short-sighted and inconsistent with sustained research and training competence.

Changing Patterns of Funding

There is, therefore, great need for public funding agencies to support the evolving role of industrialized-country research institutions. As Chapter 3 made clear, there are two main elements in the flow of funds to industrialized-country researchers for work on developing-country health problems: publicly funded research and bilateral and multilateral ODA.

Publicly funded research

Publicly funded health research in industrialized countries has grown rapidly since World War II, amounting in 1986 to about $15 billion. The major industrialized-country investors in health research are the United States, Japan, and West Germany; together they account for over

two-thirds of the total (Table 6.1). An estimated 2 percent of the total is directed at developing-country health problems, with expenditures varying among countries from under 2 percent by Japan and the United States to over 4 percent by France, Sweden, and the United Kingdom. Most public investments come from ministries of health, although additional investments often come from departments of education, foreign affairs, defense, and science and technology—agencies that operate with different priorities.

This variation among countries may be explained in part by the long-established training and technical assistance roles, frequently based on historical ties, that industrialized-country researchers have played with respect to health problems of the developing world. In general, however, most attention is focused on generating new technologies and little is targeted at improving the re-

Table 6.2 Selected international health research centers

CENTERS	ESTABLISHED	1986 BUDGET (MILLION $)	FIELD OF RESEARCH
SELECTED PAHO CENTERS			
Institute for Nutrition of Central America and Panama, Guatemala City, Guatemala (INCAP)	1946	6.6	Nutrition
Caribbean Food and Nutrition Institute, University of West Indies, Jamaica (CFNI)	1967		Nutrition
Caribbean Epidemiology Center, Port-of-Spain, Trinidad (CAREC)	1975	2.8	Disease surveillance
Pan American Center for Sanitary Engineering and Environmental Sciences, Lima, Peru (CEPIS)	1968	2.5	Environmental health
FRANCOPHONE PROGRAMS			
Organisation de Coordination et de Coopération pour la Lutte contre les Grandes Endémies en Afrique Centrale, Yaounde, Cameroon (OCEAC)	—	0.9*	Endemic diseases
Organisation de Coordination et de Coopération pour la Lutte contre les Grandes Endémies, Burkina-Faso (OCCGE)	—	3.9*	Endemic diseases
OTHER CENTERS			
International Agency for Research on Cancer, Lyons, France (IARC)	1965	8.5	Cancer
International Centre for Diarrhoeal Disease Research, Bangladesh, Dhaka (ICDDR,B)	1978	7.7	Diarrheal disease

*Shows contributions from the French government only.   Source: Commission survey

search capacity of developing countries.

Bilateral and multilateral ODA

The strategy of ODA support for industrialized-country research and education varies among donor countries. In some cases, explicit efforts are made by ODA agencies to strengthen the capability of home-country institutions to contribute to health research on developing-country problems. A more common pattern is for industrialized-country groups to be considered operational arms of ODA agencies and asked to undertake technical assistance and servicing functions.

For both domestic public research funding agencies and ODA agencies, there is a great need for the type of support that would provide greater financial stability and research training for industrialized-country groups to attract and retain able young researchers. Support is needed also to provide career structures for industrialized-country groups so that they can contribute to capacity building of developing-country researchers and participate in regional and international networking arrangements. A culture of partnership can be developed only if sufficient resources are made available to enable industrialized-country groups to participate appropriately.

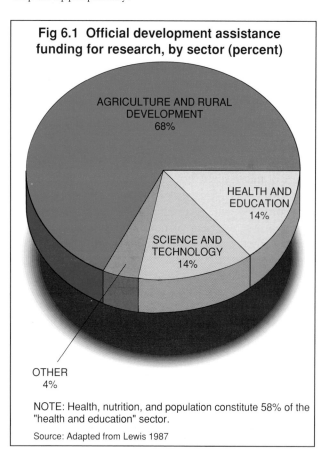

Fig 6.1 Official development assistance funding for research, by sector (percent)

AGRICULTURE AND RURAL DEVELOPMENT
68%

HEALTH AND EDUCATION
14%

SCIENCE AND TECHNOLOGY
14%

OTHER
4%

NOTE: Health, nutrition, and population constitute 58% of the "health and education" sector.

Source: Adapted from Lewis 1987

International Centers

International centers play an important role in health research. Yet sharp differences of opinion exist within the international health community as to their appropriateness and effectiveness. On the one hand, internationally organized efforts have the advantage of achieving a critical mass of scientists concentrating on and physically situated close to high-priority problems. Consequently, such efforts should be able to generate high-quality research in the short run. Moreover, internationally organized research efforts can focus on specific problems in a multidisciplinary way and demonstrate economies of scale in their operations, making them attractive to external funders.

On the other hand, international center salaries are high, and their modes of operation are expensive; their activities, if not carefully targeted, can supersede rather than complement national efforts. Although international efforts may generate high-quality research quickly, the relevance of this research to priority needs of a host country may be questionable. Moreover, salary disparities between foreign and local staff have repeatedly generated management difficulties at some centers, compromising their productivity.

Several international health research centers—an illustrative number of which are listed in Table 6.2 (page 57)—have developed over the past several decades. The first four centers listed in the table are the largest of some 10 centers established and supported by PAHO in the Americas. The second group listed involves Francophone countries in Central (OCEAC) and Western (OCCGE) Africa. The last two centers listed are the largest of the international centers. IARC, based in France, is a WHO center for international cancer research, and ICDDR,B, in Bangladesh, is an independent center that pursues research on the diarrheal diseases.

International centers in the field of health are few and small compared to those that have been developed in the field of agriculture. It is thus useful to review the agricultural experience for possible lessons.

Lessons from Agriculture

Two important functions are performed by the organized and coordinated international effort in the field of agricultural research. The first is research on food crops and related subjects, conducted in 13 international centers. The second is overall assessment of research progress and needs, and promotion of appropriate action, including resource mobilization, performed by the Consultative Group on International Agricultural Research (CGIAR). In summary, while we believe that international research centers have more limited usefulness in the field of health than in agriculture, we also believe that a health analogue of the CGIAR assessment and promotion structure could be of great value and should be established.

Research on the agricultural needs of developing countries has been assisted since the mid-1960s by a network of 13 international agricultural research centers, the earliest and most distinguished of which are the International Maize and Wheat Center (CIMMYT) in Mexico and the International Rice Research Institute (IRRI) in the Philippines. All 13 are sponsored, staffed, managed, and financed on an international basis. Ten focus on specific food crops and three pursue special functions: international food policy (IFPRI), strengthening national research systems (ISNAR), and the preservation of germ plasm (IBPGR).

The international centers are monitored, reviewed, and supported by the CGIAR, which has a small secretariat housed at the World Bank in Washington, D.C. The CGIAR includes representatives of international agencies, donor agencies, and developing countries. The CGIAR facilitates investment decisions by the donors based upon regular needs assessments and research evaluations by a Technical Advisory Committee (TAC), which is served by its own small secretariat based at the Food and Agriculture Organization (FAO) in Rome. Currently the CGIAR is considering the possible addition of several centers to the 13 it now sponsors. Donors are reportedly pleased with the efficiency and effectiveness of the CGIAR mechanism, although critics charge that the system does not possess sufficient developing-country participation in decision-making and that the international research centers have not made adequate

contributions to the development of national research capacity.

The CGIAR mechanism has been so successful in mobilizing resources that it commands about one-third of total external funding for agricultural research in developing countries. A recent study suggested that agriculture receives about two-thirds of the research aid of five major bilateral donors, compared to less than 9 percent allocated for the health field (Figure 6.1). Repeatedly, the question has arisen whether similar arrangements might help accelerate health research; whether a CGIAR/TAC-international-centers model should be crafted for the health field. In addressing this issue, we find it useful to distinguish two questions. Should autonomous international centers be developed in the health field? Are there other attributes of the CGIAR that could be adapted to suit the needs of the health field?

On balance, we consider that while some research functions may be better performed in international centers, the establishment of new international health research centers would not be the most effective and economical way to proceed at present. Rather, it would be preferable to direct resources toward strengthening existing and new national research centers in developing countries and linking these centers in international networks with some division of labor. This should provide for the development of the strongest national centers to serve both national and international purposes such as advanced training and leadership in collaborative research. In one illustration of a possible combination of national and international purposes, the Pan American Health Organization is exploring establishing in the Caribbean and Latin America a regional system for research and development on vaccines, including two subregional centers and 10 affiliated laboratories (Box 6.5).

It will not be easy to build national centers to the degree of strength required to serve international purposes and with the necessary degree of responsiveness to international as well as national needs. Nevertheless, we believe such an approach is appropriate to our present historical period and to accustomed methods of health research. Existing international centers that address high-priority problems should continue to be supported, and new centers should be considered on a case-by-case basis when judged essential for addressing global health problems that require a focused international effort.

On the other hand, we view the CGIAR and TAC mechanisms as highly relevant to the needs of the health field. The functions of maintaining a global overview across many specific health problems backed by independent technical assessments and the capacity to mobilize resources in support of larger research efforts are sorely missing. Provided there is ample developing-country representation in the decision-making process, analogues to the CGIAR and the TAC could be extremely constructive for the health field.

Conclusions

1. Industrialized-country researchers and research institutions contribute substantially to research on health problems of developing countries. However, the vicissitudes of funding and institutional support are limiting recruitment and career development of young scientists and research output. In light of the growing global interdependence in health, the interests of both industrialized and developing countries would be well served by strengthening and stabilizing support for these institutions.

2. Priorities and patterns of institutional develop-

ment in industrialized countries have favored and supported excellent biomedical research but have neglected policy, management, economics, behavioral, and social research. This not only constrains the research done in industrialized countries but also diminishes its relevance for developing countries.

3. Health research institutions in industrialized countries should seek collaborative arrangements with their counterparts in developing countries for collegial exchange and training, capacity building, and research. Industrialized-country groups should participate in regional and international networks.

4. Funding agencies need to adjust their policies to support appropriate and sustained development of domestic institutions engaged in research on Third World health problems. Short-term, one-way technical assistance, episodic project activities, and other forms of support should be balanced with stronger, longer-term support for capacity building, two-way exchange, and other partnership arrangements by industrialized groups in their work with developing-country counterparts.

5. For the health field, international functions can be better achieved by strengthening national institutions within developing countries to play both national and international roles, buttressed by regional and international networking, rather than by creating new autonomous international health research centers. Existing international centers should continue to be supported, and the possibility of new ones should be kept under review if needed for special purposes.

6. An international facilitation mechanism for health research, similar to the Consultative Group for International Agricultural Research, should be established. This would bring greater coherence to support for research on health problems of developing countries, and also would have the potential of mobilizing greater long-term funding in support of such research.

CHAPTER 7

International Research Promotion

D istinct from researchers and institutions that conduct research, like those reviewed in the previous two chapters, are agencies and programs that promote health research undertaken by others through funding, mobilizing, directing, and supporting researchers and their institutions.[1] Some of these programs also focus on building and sustaining research capacity in developing countries. Although their financing is usually international—as are their patterns of research collaboration, technical interaction, and communications—they can and do play a critical role in nurturing country-specific as well as global research activities throughout the world.

The past two decades have witnessed a significant expansion of international research promotion programs. Consequently, the beginnings of a worldwide health research system with many component parts is emerging. These promotional activities and their organizational bases—the UN system, private initiatives, bilateral aid, and private industry—are the subject of this chapter.

The United Nations System

Of the many participants in research promotion, the most significant is the World Health Organization. With an annual budget of about $500 million and a staff of nearly 5,000 based in its Geneva headquarters, six regional offices, and country offices around the world, WHO is the principal intergovernmental organization for health.

The WHO charter gives the organization a mandate "to promote and conduct research in the field of health." Funds for research constitute only a small proportion (less than 2 percent) of WHO's regular budget. However, research activities associated with WHO and supported by extrabudgetary funds have grown markedly in the last two decades. Total research funded from both regular and extra-budgetary sources rose to more than $60 million per year in the 1980s (Figure 7.1). Most of the research is devoted to specific diseases (tropical disease, diarrhea, AIDS) and to protecting the health of specific population groups (maternal and child health and reproductive health) (Figure 7.2).

A highly complex organization, WHO conducts little research itself but promotes research in connection with many of its offices and programs. Responsibili-

> *Developing countries must build up their own basis for research. Only they will be able to establish the diagnosis and implement the cure. The international community must assist the process.*
>
> **Gro Harlem Brundtland**
> *Chair, the World Commission on Environment and Development*

ty for coordinating research in WHO is assigned to an Office for Research Promotion and Development (ORPD), which also services the Advisory Committee on Health Research (ACHR). The ACHR advises the director-general of WHO on research matters, providing broad oversight on health research within and beyond the agency. Regional ACHRs perform similar functions for WHO's six regional directors.

WHO-associated Research

As noted, the great bulk of WHO funding for research comes from extrabudgetary resources, mobilized from public and private donors for a series of programs that address high-priority global health problems. These programs vary considerably in size, organizational pattern, and research focus. The largest are the Special Programme of Research, Development, and Research Training in Human Reproduction (HRP), begun in 1972, and the Special Programme for Research and Training in Tropical Diseases (TDR), begun in 1976 (Box 7.1, page 64). Together, these two programs disburse about $40-50 million annually for research projects and for strengthening research capacity in developing countries—about

two-thirds of WHO's annual spending for research.

The HRP and TDR programs are jointly sponsored by WHO and other UN agencies (UNDP, World Bank, and, in the case of HRP, UNFPA) and governed by special boards, with WHO acting as the host and manager of the programs' day-to-day affairs. Their primary focus is on finding new knowledge and technologies for dealing with human reproduction and with six selected tropical diseases: malaria, schistosomiasis, filariasis, trypanosomiasis, leishmaniasis, and leprosy. Both programs operate through scientific working groups made up of leading scientists from developing and industrialized countries. The working groups define priority research agendas and distribute available funds to high-priority, quality research projects around the world.

Other substantial WHO-affiliated research programs are those of the Onchocerciasis Control Programme (OCP), the Programme for Control of Diarrhoeal Diseases (CDD), the Expanded Programme on Immunization (EPI), and the Global Programme on AIDS (GPA). Unlike HRP and TDR, which are exclusively focused on research and training, these other programs are organized within WHO's regular structure and promote disease-control action as well as research.

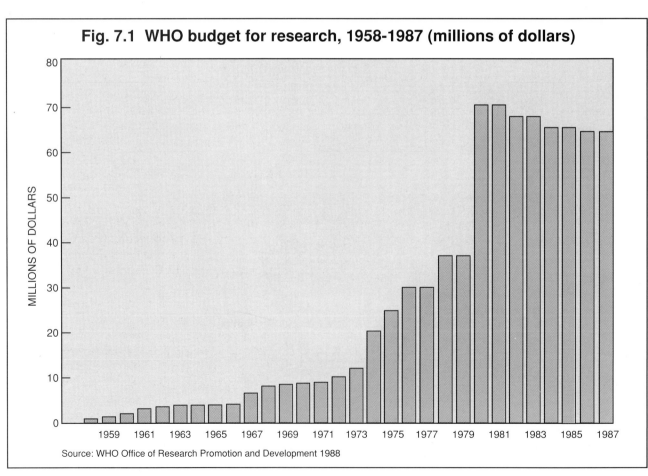

Fig. 7.1 WHO budget for research, 1958-1987 (millions of dollars)

Source: WHO Office of Research Promotion and Development 1988

OCP was established in 1974, under the regional office of WHO for Africa, as a multinational effort to control river blindness in West Africa. OCP has an active research program in support of its interventions (Box 7.2, page 65).

Established in 1978, CDD's mandate is primarily to promote action for controlling the diarrheal diseases. Its principal research activities are vaccine and drug development. Recently a new, parallel program on acute respiratory infections was established under the same leadership as CDD.

EPI is a program to promote the rapid spread of vaccination for children against measles, whooping cough, diphtheria, and other diseases for which effective vaccines exist. It carries out operations research concerned with improving the methods for achieving higher vaccination rates, measuring coverage, and evaluating results.

GPA is the most recent and fastest growing action-research program, with a budget expected to approach $100 million by 1990. Since it began only in 1986, the nature and size of its research promotion work have yet to be fully defined.

The WHO-associated research programs, especially HRP and TDR, have introduced innovations on an international scale. They have mobilized scientific talent from around the world, encouraged the participation of scientists in setting the research agenda, and fostered peer review, external independent evaluation, and accountability to donors. They have added substantially to the international effort to promote health research, but they cover only a limited range of the health problems of developing countries, and their efforts to build research capacity in developing countries are not broad-based but principally confined to their problem-focused mandates.

Other UN Agencies

Other agencies within the UN family also play a significant role in research promotion. UNICEF, concerned with the welfare of children, is primarily an operational agency supported by voluntary contributions, but it has increasingly supported field evaluations and assessments and the development of health information systems to support management decisions. These activities, which fall within the Commission's definition of country-specific health research, constitute about 2 per-

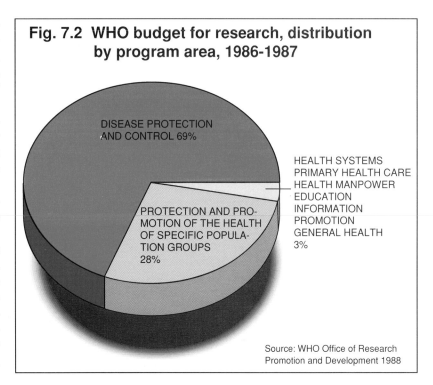

Fig. 7.2 WHO budget for research, distribution by program area, 1986-1987

DISEASE PROTECTION AND CONTROL 69%

HEALTH SYSTEMS PRIMARY HEALTH CARE HEALTH MANPOWER EDUCATION INFORMATION PROMOTION GENERAL HEALTH 3%

PROTECTION AND PROMOTION OF THE HEALTH OF SPECIFIC POPULATION GROUPS 28%

Source: WHO Office of Research Promotion and Development 1988

cent of UNICEF's overall expenditures.

The United Nations Development Programme (UNDP) is a multisectoral development agency that also supports health research, usually in cooperation with other UN agencies through its interregional program office. Currently UNDP commits over $16 million annually to health research and operates as a joint sponsor of the WHO-associated research programs described earlier. Its critical role as a broad development agency providing the link between the health sector and overall development offers substantial opportunities not yet fully realized.

UNFPA also supports research, primarily in the areas of demography, family planning, maternal and child health, and contraceptive technology. As a fund rather than a technical or operating agency, UNFPA makes grants to governments or to technical agencies of the UN system. It is a major supporter of demographic and statistical data-collection by developing countries, a core sponsor and funder of HRP, and a major participant in the support of integrated maternal-child health and family planning programs around the world.

The World Bank also jointly sponsors, and in some cases financially supports, research. It is a contributor to WHO-associated research programs. In addition, the Bank supports an internal, policy-oriented research program. As a financial institution, the Bank's research focuses on economic policy in the population, health, and nutrition sectors.

In addition to the above organizations, the UN

system includes many advisory and coordinating committees. One example is the UN Administrative Committee on Coordination—Subcommittee on Nutrition (UN ACC/SCN), which coordinates and promotes nutrition action and research in the UN system. The ACC/SCN has generated many useful reports but does not appear to have had major influence on policy and implementation. Nutrition research and action within the UN suffers from the problem of "everybody's business is nobody's business," receiving little direct attention. Although they are plainly useful, such committees do not control a research budget and have not had strong or-

---

Box 7.1 Two WHO-associated research programs: HRP and TDR

The two oldest and largest of the WHO-associated research programs are the Special Programme of Research, Development and Research Training in Human Reproduction (HRP) and the Special Programme for Research and Training in Tropical Diseases (TDR). The trend of their budgets is shown in the chart—rising at the end of the 1970s, falling back somewhat in the 1980s, and currently rising again.

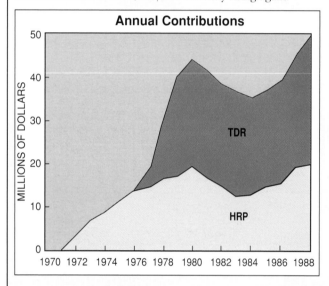

Annual Contributions

HRP began in 1972 and is co-sponsored by UNDP, UNFPA, World Bank, and WHO. Its objectives are: 1) *research and development* aimed at increased knowledge about human reproduction, including new and improved contraceptives; and 2) *research capability strengthening* through training in biomedical and social sciences and support of institutions, to raise the capability of developing countries to undertake research on fertility, infertility, sexually transmitted diseases, and other aspects of reproductive health.

HRP operates through task forces—multinational and multidisciplinary groups of scientists addressing key issues of contraceptive development and use, such as safety and efficacy, behavioral and social determinants, long-acting systemic agents, and vaccines. In addition to experimental research projects aimed at improving existing methods and finding or developing new ones, HRP works with a network of centers conducting clinical research. Over the years, the clinical research they have done has involved about 160 collaborating centers in 210 multicenter trials with a total of

220,000 patients in 55 countries.

In the years 1972-89, total contributions to HRP were $265 million, of which about one-third was spent on institution-strengthening.

Co-sponsored by UNDP, the World Bank, and WHO, **TDR** became operational in 1976, with two specific objectives: 1) *research and development* aimed at new and improved tools for the control of major tropical diseases—drugs, vaccines, diagnostic tools, and new methods for controlling the vectors of these diseases; and 2) *research capability strengthening* through training in biomedical and social sciences, and through support of institutions, to strengthen the capability of developing countries to undertake research on major tropical diseases.

Six diseases were selected for attack—malaria, schistosomiasis, filariasis (including onchocerciasis), trypanosomiases (African sleeping sickness, Chagas' disease), leishmaniasis, and leprosy. These diseases were selected on the basis of their public health importance and because existing technologies were judged to be inadequate for bringing them under control.

The program brings together researchers from a variety of biomedical and social sciences in a goal-oriented multidisciplinary attack. It mobilizes the powerful tools of modern biology—immunology, molecular biology, and biochemistry—in the search for new technologies, and it seeks collaboration with other research efforts in academia and industry around the world.

The program is managed by committees of scientists, drawn from institutions all over the world, who assess the needs and identify the most promising approaches. The program set out not to create new institutions but instead to utilize and strengthen existing ones. Research is carried out by networks of scientists, each working in an established institution.

At the end of the first 10 years, an External Review Committee noted the program's "considerable record of accomplishments." The committee observed that the program had made significant contributions to the research on some 60 products which were in use or at advanced stages of development.

On the capacity strengthening side, the program had awarded several hundred individual training grants; sponsored 13 M.Sc. training courses in epidemiology and community health, medical entomology, health economics, and parasitology; and provided various types of support to over 90 institutions in developing countries.

ganizational or financial impact in advancing research on developing-country health problems.

Private Foundations and Programs

Although their overall financial contributions are modest, private foundations have played a critical role in health research. Based primarily in North America but growing in Western Europe and Japan, private foundations invest relatively heavily in health research. As a group, they concentrate their investments in population, tropical and infectious diseases, and health policy and management (Figure 7.3, page 66). Foundations support developing-country health research primarily through grants to multilateral and industrialized-country institutions. About one-third of foundation investments in this field are granted directly to developing-country scientists and institutions.

Private foundations, because of their flexibility and independence, often identify neglected topics, pioneer the development of structures that attract larger public resources, and sometimes sustain commitment for a long period. They are also in a position to encourage nonprofit, nongovernmental participation in research, especially by private action agencies in developing countries. Their resources are relatively small and are best used to mobilize the broader support necessary for decisive attacks on major problems that require health research.

The major program concerns of nine foundations in health and population are compared in Table 7.1 (page 66). For example, MacArthur funds tropical disease research and women's health; Pew targets health policy and management; Clark, Sasakawa, and Wellcome all target tropical diseases.

The foundations often support specially designed programs as instruments of their grantmaking. For example, the South-South reproductive biology research network, funded by the Rockefeller Foundation, fosters international research cooperation among developing-country scientists on population issues. Similarly designed programs in epidemiology and health policy are the International Clinical Epidemiology Network (IN-CLEN) initiated by the Rockefeller Foundation, the International Health Policy Program (IHPP) initiated by the Pew Trusts and the Carnegie Corporation, and the Community Epidemiology and Management Networks in India and Indonesia supported by the Ford Foundation.

The activities of autonomous institutes also fill research gaps. The International Planned Parenthood Federation (IPPF), headquartered in London, serves population and reproductive health interests. Three of the more prominent institutes in North America are the Population

Box 7.2 Research on onchocerciasis

Onchocerciasis is a parasitic disease that causes eye damage and, in severe cases, blindness. WHO estimates that 86 million people in the developing world are at risk from the disease, which is most severe in the savannah areas of West Africa. The Onchocerciasis Control Programme (OCP) was set up in 1974 at the request of seven West African countries (Benin, Burkina Faso, Ivory Coast, Ghana, Mali, Niger, and Togo). In 1986, four more countries (Guinea, Guinea-Bissau, Senegal, and Sierra Leone) joined. Supported by a group of 23 donor countries and international agencies, OCP now covers an area containing about 30 million persons.

In humans infected with onchocerciasis, parasites are present both as adult worms and as microscopic larvae, microfilariae. During a lifespan of about 11 years, the adult female produces millions of microfilariae that live about 30 months, during which time they migrate through the body. Dead microfilariae under the skin cause an inflammatory response that produces the main symptoms of onchocerciasis.

The disease is transmitted by a black fly that breeds near fast-flowing streams. The OCP strategy has been to attack the vulnerable fly larvae through serial application of insecticides to thousands of breeding sites. After 15 years of vector control, transmission of the disease has been controlled in large parts of the original area covered by the program. In 80 percent of this area, the human reservoir of the parasite has been virtually eliminated, and vector control operations will cease in 1990. In the next decade OCP will continue larviciding areas to the south and west of the original area in order to prevent reinvasion by migrating flies and to control transmission of the disease until the reservoir of adult parasites has died out in human hosts.

Along with its strong operational focus, OCP has conducted substantial research ranging from laboratory to ecological investigations. An applied research program was launched in 1974, and in 1982, OCP set up an Onchocerciasis Chemotherapy Unit under the technical supervision of TDR, with the purpose of funding research to identify a macrofilaricide capable of killing adult worms. On average, about 12 percent of OCP's total costs has been spent on research.

With the development of ivermectin by the American pharmaceutical firm Merck, Sharp and Dohme, and in collaboration with TDR/OCP, an effective and safe microfilaricide was produced. Tested in the field from 1987 to 1989, ivermectin is now being distributed in highly endemic areas. Ivermectin enhances OCP's effectiveness by providing it with the means to deal quickly with severe effects of onchocerciasis in heavily infected populations. However, OCP estimates that ivermectin use alone will not suffice to control transmission. Further research, including investigations of immunodiagnostic tests and macrofilaricides, is needed.

Council, the Program for Applied Technology in Health (PATH), and Family Health International (FHI). These autonomous policy, research, and action agencies undertake a substantial amount of direct research as well as research promotion in their fields of specialization.

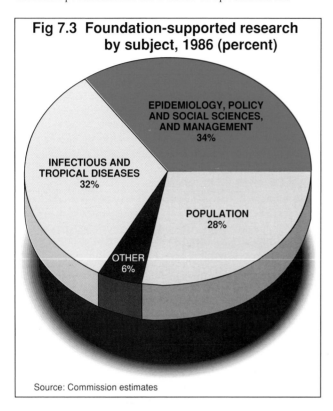

Fig 7.3 Foundation-supported research by subject, 1986 (percent)

EPIDEMIOLOGY, POLICY AND SOCIAL SCIENCES, AND MANAGEMENT 34%

INFECTIOUS AND TROPICAL DISEASES 32%

POPULATION 28%

OTHER 6%

Source: Commission estimates

Table 7.1 Foundation programs related to international health and population

Foundation	Program focus
Aga Khan Foundation	Management of primary health care
Carnegie Corporation	Strengthening human resources
Edna McConnell Clark Foundation	Tropical disease research
Ford Foundation	Reproductive health
MacArthur Foundation	Tropical health; parasitic diseases; women's health networks
Pew Charitable Trusts	Health policy and management
Rockefeller Foundation	Great neglected diseases; INCLEN; population sciences
Sasakawa Memorial Health Foundation	Leprosy eradication
Wellcome Trust	Medical and veterinary research

Sources: Foundation annual reports 1985-87

Most nongovernmental organizations—especially private voluntary agencies such as CARE, Save the Children, Oxfam, and the Red Cross—are action-oriented. Research usually plays only a minor role, but several have active research programs to support their activities and have made significant contributions, especially in areas concerned with the health of refugees and disaster victims, community-based health, and health information.

Special Research Agencies

The International Development Research Centre of Canada (IDRC) and the Swedish Agency for Research in Developing Countries (SAREC) are publicly supported, semi-autonomous development-research funding agencies whose strategies and approaches more closely parallel those of private foundations than those of governmental foreign assistance agencies. IDRC has substantial developing-country representation on its board of governors and a network of regional field offices for direct grantmaking overseas. SAREC similarly encourages developing-country researchers, often linked with Swedish counterparts. IDRC and SAREC are particularly noteworthy for their strong emphasis on the role of the social sciences in health research.

Bilateral ODA

Bilateral development assistance agencies have the greatest potential to support health research through their aid projects or through grants to intermediary organizations. Considerable support has in fact been channeled by bilateral agencies through the WHO-associated research programs. However, most bilateral agencies have provided little support directly to developing countries for health research and research capacity building. This may be caused by their preference for action over research, and by lack of time and expert staff to appraise relatively small components in health projects or separate research projects.

In view of the importance of the results of country-specific health research to the design, implementation, and evaluation of health projects, there is a strong case for bilateral agencies to include routinely a research component in every health project. Some aid agencies, notably the U.S. Agency for International Development, have experimented successfully with using knowledgeable independent sources to assist in appraising and funding research components and research projects. These methods may yield more useful research results, but further innovations will be required to pro-

Box 7.3 Industry collaboration in research on developing-country health problems

There is great need to promote pharmaceutical industry participation in and support of research on developing-country health problems. One positive development within industry has been its collaboration with multilateral organizations. The TDR program, for example, has established a working exchange with pharmaceutical companies to encourage the inclusion of developing-country health priorities within industry research agendas. Industry collaboration with TDR in 1987-88 generated many activities, among them:

• development of new formulations of *Bacillus thuringiensis H-14* and *B. sphaericus* that control the insect vectors of tropical diseases (Abbott Laboratories, United States);

• development and testing of macrofilaricides for the treatment of onchocerciasis and lymphatic filariasis (Ciba-Geigy Limited, Switzerland);

• development and testing of mefloquine for the treatment of malaria (F. Hoffman-LaRoche and Co., United States);

• testing of halofantrine for the treatment of malaria (Smith, Kline and French Laboratories, United States);

• development of new formulations for controlling the insect vectors of tropical diseases (Solvay et Cie., Belgium/Duphar B.V., Netherlands);

• double-blind trials with reduced dosages of melarsoprol for African trypanosomiasis (SPECIA, France);

In addition to the commitment of research and development *resources* to health problems affecting developing countries, commitment of research *products* characterizes a desirable model of pharmaceutical-company collaboration. An outstanding example of this is Merck's recent donation of ivermectin to combat onchocerciasis, the cause of river blindness.

In general, however, the pharmaceutical industry responds to market forces in developing new and improved drugs. The incentive structure drives product development toward those drugs for which there is a market. The cost of developing a new drug today is an estimated $100 million. Fresh mechanisms that promote incentives for research on health problems of developing countries (such as front-end funding mechanisms, highlighted in Box 7.5) as well as measures to monitor the relationship between pharmaceutical companies and the developing world, can produce still greater benefits and can cement stronger collaborative relationships between pharmaceutical companies and developing-country interests.

---

vide the sustained support necessary to build research capacity in developing countries.

Private Industry

The pharmaceutical industry has one of the highest levels of research and development investment of all commercial fields. But pharmaceutical companies find very little incentive to develop products for markets where purchasing power is limited, as is the case in the poorer developing countries. However, some private industry collaborative activities are already underway with the WHO-associated research programs, particularly in clinical and field testing of new technologies (Box 7.3).

Convincing pharmaceutical companies to research and develop products for less lucrative markets will not be easy. New pharmaceuticals now cost an average of over $100 million to develop, and the process may take 10 years or longer. Technologies such as contraceptives and vaccines have high-liability risks in litigious societies. Adding to the problems is the growing international controversy over proprietary rights and access to new information and technologies (Box 7.4, page 68). In the face of these challenges, new incentives may be required, such as the Child Survival Task Force's strategy for encouraging industry to join in vaccine production through assurances regarding front-end funding

(Box 7.5, page 68). In view of the hazards arising from the widespread misuse of drugs such as antibiotics, the pharmaceutical industry might be induced to support a research program to promote the rational use of therapeutic drugs.

The Need for an Overview Mechanism

The complex worldwide system for promoting health research on health and development lacks an effective overview mechanism. While the determinants of ill health and its consequences for development are broad, the dominant perspective among those who fund health research remains a medical one. Most existing mechanisms, such as the WHO-associated research programs, are narrowly targeted, and the information needed to gain a perspective encompassing the full breadth of health and development is fragmentary or unavailable. Overall, the promotional programs appear to have been more successful in promoting global research than country-specific research. Moreover, international programs aimed at single problems possess inherent weaknesses in building national scientific and institutional capacity.

The various agencies described in this chapter make important contributions to worldwide health research, but significant gaps remain. The ACHR has the

Box 7.4 Debate over intellectual property rights

Access to intellectual advances is vital to the progress of all societies, developing and industrialized. Yet 97 percent of research and development of all forms is carried out in high-income countries. The UN Commission on Trade and Development estimates that the number of scientists, engineers, and technicians engaged in R&D in developing countries is less than 1.5 per 10,000 inhabitants, compared with 16.6 in the industrialized market economies.

The rights to intellectual property, including the fruits of health research, have become a contentious issue. The debate is likely to remain at the forefront of international negotiations due to the growing share of intellectual property in international trade and also because of inherent conceptual, legal, and diplomatic complexities. For developing countries, access to intellectual property, especially technological and scientific products, is essential. Monopolistic charges for these products may place them out of reach in an overall economic climate of declining foreign investment, international indebtedness, and protectionism in industrial-

ized-country markets. Developing countries must strengthen their scientific and technological capabilities, overcome global imbalances, and advance their own development.

The primary producers of new technological and scientific products are private industry, research institutes, and universities in North America, Europe, and Japan. Advocates of internationally applicable intellectual property rights argue that protection is needed to offset the cost of R&D, to yield profit for investments, and to provide an incentive for future innovation. The cost of R&D required to create new products is increasing, while the number of relevant new products may be decreasing.

The debate on intellectual property rights is likely to continue. Ultimate resolution depends upon the long-term development of R&D capabilities more balanced between the developing and the industrialized countries, and on reconciling the competing interests of economic incentives and rewards for innovation with the need for equitable health and development worldwide.

---

advantage of operating within WHO as the nodal point of transdisease and transdivisional perspectives on health research. However, while ACHR's reports are generally useful, the committee has a restricted mandate, little promotional role, no budget, and only an advisory function to WHO. It does not involve the other UN agencies concerned with health and development, and it has been dominated by biomedical scientists. The regional ACHRs are often tied to national medical research councils and ministries of health, reinforcing the predominantly medical focus. In addition, the ACHRs meet infrequently, in some regions only every other year.

It is difficult to escape the conclusion that the current system of promoting research on developing-country health problems is fragmented and lacks overall co-

herence. No mechanism exists currently to identify and promote research on problems that lack an advocacy group. There is no mechanism to deal with the normal, difficult questions of rationalizing global research efforts, for example: Which problems deserve more attention? Which less? When is a problem "solved"? There is no institutional memory for research. What lessons are being learned? How are these lessons informing other initiatives? Individual international research programs, such as TDR, HRP, CDD, and ICDDR,B, are separately evaluated regularly, but there is no ongoing mechanism whereby the results of these evaluations are used to inform the general process of international health research and development. And there is no independent, informal voice to speak frankly and critically on the policies and practices of agencies. It is very difficult for one in-

---

Box 7.5 Front-end funding for vaccine development

The Task Force for Child Survival—supported by WHO, UNICEF, UNDP, the World Bank, and the Rockefeller Foundation, and headquartered at the Carter Center in Atlanta (United States)—has initiated an innovative promotion scheme to ensure that new and improved vaccines will be available to people in developing countries. By offering financial assistance for vaccine development to commercial manufacturers as a means of offsetting high research costs, in exchange for lower vaccine prices, the task force hopes to speed development of selected vaccines and to enhance their affordability. This research incentive system is known as front-end funding.

The first round of proposals has been reviewed by the task force. Six submissions, each proposing an effective new

vaccine to become available to EPI in less than five years, were considered. Five of those were offered by a new consortium of the Dutch-Nordic public health institutes and one by Sclavo, an Italian vaccine manufacturing firm. The vaccines considered are to protect against meningococcus A&C, pneumococcus, cholera, Japanese encephalitis, and mininococcus B. The scientific review team gave the highest rating to the meningococcus A&C proposal of Sclavo and the pneumococcal proposal initiated by the Finnish Institute of the Dutch-Nordic group. Once technical questions raised by the reviewers have been resolved, the Task Force for Child Survival will seek resources from donor agencies. It will also negotiate for transfer of the technology to developing-world institutions.

ternational agency to comment on another's policies and unlikely that an agency or a developing country would criticize another agency on which it depends for financial support. With the evolution of a pluralistic global health research system, independent assessment and advocacy are necessary to address these deficiencies.

Conclusions

1. WHO in collaboration with other agencies has launched some highly successful health research efforts in the past two decades, which represent the beginnings of a worldwide health research system. The success of the WHO-associated research programs has shown that interagency cooperation within the UN can lead to increased investments and greater focus, coherence, and productivity. They have also demonstrated the effectiveness of a network model of research, a strategy that mobilizes scientific talent around the world. Despite these laudable efforts, major problems such as acute respiratory infections, tuberculosis, substance abuse, and country-specific health research have not received the attention they deserve.

2. Multilateral agencies such as UNICEF, UNDP, the World Bank, regional banks, and bilateral assistance agencies, all of which spend substantial sums on health projects, are important sources for additional funds to support research and networking on developing-country health problems (Box 7.6). New mechanisms may be required to provide technical review of research components and research projects for some of these agencies.

3. International research agencies (IDRC and SAREC) and private foundations, though limited in resources, have played and should continue to play valuable roles because of their independence, flexibility, capable professional staff, and ability to sustain commitments over extended periods of time.

4. The large health research resources of private industry are engaged to a distressingly small extent in research on developing-country health problems. Innovative measures should continue to be sought to promote the mobilization of more of these resources to address health problems of developing countries.

5. Overview arrangements for assessing progress in research on developing-country health problems, identifying neglected areas, and promoting necessary action are needed to ensure that resources are effectively deployed in a pluralistic worldwide health research system.

CHAPTER 8

Building and Sustaining Research Capacity

Strengthening research capacity in developing countries is one of the most powerful, cost-effective, and sustainable means of advancing health and development. The overall goal of capacity building is to improve the capabilities of individuals and institutions to address health problems through research. The concepts of country-specific and global health research can help attain this goal by providing a clear framework for setting objectives, measuring progress, determining investment priorities, and guiding actions. Capacity building should be undertaken on a country-by-country basis, adapted to the unique circumstances of each nation.

Capacity Building Defined

Building capacity for science-based development involves at least four components.[1]

1. Individual competence
Competence includes not only the skills needed to use particular disciplines, but also a systematic and scientific approach to problem solving. Thus, strengthening research capacity means strengthening those skills and attributes associated both with the direct conduct of research and with successful policy formulation and research-based management of action for health and development.

2. Institutional infrastructure that supports research
Actions in this category include upgrading career structures, salaries, scientific information, facilities, equipment, and supplies; improving research priority setting and the management of research activities; increasing training capacity; and developing operational links with action units in the country. In addition to universities and research institutes, we include ministries and departments of government, and nongovernmental organizations oriented toward action-research, as prospective sites for health research capacity building.

3. The research component of policy formulation and field action
The precise boundary between research and action is difficult to delineate.

> *It is likely that an extremely important long-term contribution of the current Health for All movement will be to establish in every country, and in every community, an evolving capacity to deal with the health problems of that place and time.*
>
> **WHO meeting at Riga, 1988**

COMMISSION ON HEALTH RESEARCH FOR DEVELOPMENT

We have adopted a broad definition of research, which considers systematic analysis of health information at one extreme to sophisticated laboratory experiments at the other as relevant objectives for research capacity strengthening.

This Commission adopted the term essential national health research (ENHR) to describe the health research—and the health research capacity—on which each developing country should concentrate. Capacity to conduct ENHR means the ability to undertake two research approaches. The first is to conduct research on country-specific health problems. Every country needs the results of such research to formulate sound policies and plans for field action. In most developing countries this kind of research capacity has been neglected, and to build it deserves highest priority. To this end, major ef-

forts are needed to strengthen epidemiology, the social sciences (particularly economics), health management, and applied clinical and biomedical research. It is also critical to create a demand for research among those responsible for policy formulation and field action. This may be fostered by good communication between research groups and the users of their results and by involving the users in setting research priorities and time schedules.

4. Global health research

The second element of ENHR for each developing country is to contribute as much as possible to research aimed at discovering new knowledge and technologies to solve health problems of significance to its population. Each country must assess its own ability to partici-

---

Box 8.1 Building capacity for demographic research in China

Over the past 15 years, a remarkable build-up has occurred in China's capacity to analyze its huge and growing population—over one billion persons, about one-fifth of the world's total. In the 1970s, when China's government recognized the urgent need for country-specific research on population trends and problems as a basis for policy and program decisions, they found themselves with virtually no Chinese demographers. Demographic training and research had been proscribed in China for about 20 years following the "hundred flowers" period of the mid-1950s.

Beginning in the late 1970s, a series of vigorous actions has been taken:

• University-based population research institutes were founded, numbering 38 by 1986. Population research units were also established in the Chinese Academy of Social Sciences, the State Planning Commission, the State Family Planning Commission, the Census Office, and other governmental bodies. There were over 50 specialized population research units by late 1985.

• An early step was to shift scholars who had been trained in other fields to population studies. The first generation of population researchers includes specialists from statistics, medicine, labor economics, geography and other disciplines—except for demography, sociology, anthropology, and other social sciences that had been suspended in the 1950s. By 1987, 26 of the university-based institutes reported a total of 473 population researchers.

• Many members of the first generation of population specialists were sent for one-year courses to the United Nations population training centers in Cairo and Bombay. A larger infusion of demographic skills will occur when the second generation, now completing full graduate training at universities in the United States and other industrialized countries, return to China. Moreover, China's population institutes themselves have recently begun to offer M.A. and Ph.D. programs.

• A lively program of publications was undertaken. By 1987 there were five journals devoted to population is-

sues, plus many limited-circulation publications such as translations, working papers, and research monographs.

• Technical assistance from the United Nations Fund for Population Activities (UNFPA) has been crucial to the rapid development of China's research centers. In 1980 the UNFPA began to provide books, micro-computers, technical advice and other assistance to 11 of the new institutes, adding assistance to 10 more in 1985 and a final two in 1987. Even with this assistance, however, China's population institutes, according to a recent review, suffer from weaknesses typical of developing countries—shortages of Western-language texts and monographs, particularly in the areas of theory and techniques, and of data-processing, photocopying, and other equipment necessary to operate an efficient research center.

The Chinese experience demonstrates important lessons. When a nation's leadership, even in very low-income countries, determines that capacity for country-specific research is essential and commits the necessary energy and resources, results can come with impressive speed. In China's case, an initial set of population institutes was established in both universities and governments; an initial staff was gathered by shifting people trained in other fields; and initial programs of research, training, and publication were started, all within a decade. By many accounts, the results have already been substantially beneficial in clarifying and modifying China's population policies.

Nevertheless, remarkable as the achievements thus far have been, they are only a partial answer to China's needs. Full demographic training for researchers is only now being completed. Considering the time that will still be required for them to embark on effective research careers and to begin rising into leadership positions, it will have taken approximately two decades to build a set of research and training institutions in China that are fully qualified to analyze China's population situation, to offer policy advice, and to interpret China's extraordinary population evolution to the world.

Box 8.2 Newer foundation programs to support capacity building

The philanthropic community worldwide is a significant source of support for health research in the developing world. Several new philanthropic efforts illustrate roles in supporting the development of individual and institutional capacity.

The **Aga Khan Foundation**, established in Switzerland in 1967, focuses primarily on education, health, and rural development in Pakistan, Bangladesh, India, Kenya, and Tanzania. The foundation places heavy emphasis on building competence at the community level, through the training of individuals and development of institutions that will enable community groups to analyze their own problems and to deal with them. One noteworthy project is the Aga Khan Rural Support Programme, which is working in three districts in the high mountain areas of Chitral, Gilgit, and Baltistan in northern Pakistan to establish village-based agricultural and irrigation projects, schools, and health activities. To date, over 1,000 village organizations have been established, serving a total population of about 800,000.

The **Sasakawa Memorial Health Foundation**, established in Japan in 1974, focuses primarily on support of research and action against leprosy. Working mainly in East and Southeast Asia, Sasakawa builds both individual and institutional research capacity. The foundation's capacity-building activities include sponsorship of international meetings focused on leprosy research and action; construction of the Sasakawa Memorial Research Building, part of Raj-Pracha-Samasi Institute in Bangkok, Thailand, a leprosy chemotherapy research center; and support of the Sasakawa Foundation Fellowships and Scholarships to support leprosy researchers and workers at a variety of levels. By 1987 approximately 370 fellowships and scholarships had been awarded to individuals from East and Southeast Asian countries in which leprosy is endemic.

The **Pew Charitable Trusts** represent seven individual charitable funds established between 1948 and 1979. The trusts support nonprofit activities in seven broad categories, including health. International funding within this category has begun in recent years; it is focused primarily on strengthening developing countries' capacity to address the critical health and development needs of their people. Grants support policy research and education and training programs that improve the allocation of existing resources and the delivery of services to those most in need, especially high-risk groups such as women and children and refugee populations.

Box 8.3 Research capacity building by IDRC and SAREC

Developing countries should be able to create their own health research agendas, but their ability to do so has been jeopardized by their heavy reliance on external aid. In partial response to this problem, research development agencies such as IDRC (International Development Research Centre, Canada) and SAREC (Swedish Agency for Research Cooperation with Developing Countries) have committed themselves to supporting developing-country researchers and to strengthening research capacity in developing countries.

IDRC was established by the Parliament of Canada in 1970 as an autonomous public corporation to stimulate and support research in the developing world. It concentrates its efforts in the fields of agriculture, health, communications, earth and engineering sciences, and social sciences. Although IDRC support is channeled primarily through particular research projects, the strengthening of research capacity is seen as an essential outcome of this approach.

Experience has shown IDRC that an emphasis on projects alone may leave crucial gaps in national research capacity. Therefore, institutional and program support and small grants programs are used to complement project support. IDRC field staff help grantees address technical and research management needs through workshops, networks, and formal and informal training. Linkages and exchanges with scientists in other developing countries working in similar fields are important to IDRC's policy of fostering greater indigenous control and development.

IDRC recently re-examined the role of institution building, concluding that systematic attention to institutional needs and potential can have a very high payoff. IDRC's Health Sciences Division currently devotes 30 percent of its funds to long-term institutional support.

SAREC was founded in 1975 and has had the status of an independent Swedish government agency since 1979. Its main objective is to support endogenous research that is particularly relevant to the problems of development. To achieve this, SAREC concentrates its research support in the fields of agriculture, health, technology, energy, and the social sciences, and actively encourages Swedish collaboration with researchers in the developing world. Agricultural (including environmental) research and health research account for about 70 percent of the budget allocations. Although SAREC originally allocated 90 percent of its budget to international research programs, this level of support had by 1989 dropped to less than 40 percent, allowing SAREC to devote an increasing proportion of its funds to national and regional research.

While there is no one correct method to promote research in the developing world, the experiences of IDRC and SAREC have demonstrated the importance of systematic strengthening of national research capacity. Their kind of long-term, flexible funding strategy offers developing countries the opportunity to achieve a greater degree of autonomy in their research efforts on both country-specific and global health problems.

Box 8.4 Building epidemiological and field research capacities: the TDR experience

From its beginning, the strengthening of research capabilities in countries where tropical diseases are endemic has been a major objective of the Special Programme for Research and Training in Tropical Disease Research (TDR). In the first 10 years the strategy emphasized selecting the most advanced institutions and strengthening them as needed to achieve a reasonable degree of research self-sufficiency. During this time nearly 100 institutions received support and almost 600 scientists obtained training fellowships from TDR.

In the past two years, TDR has launched a new phase. Although all aspects of research capacity in the endemic countries require strengthening, epidemiological and field research capabilities have been the weakest components and pose the greatest challenges. New initiatives include the following:

• Research training will be carried out in the context of ongoing research whenever possible. The shift in support from master's level training toward the doctoral level will continue; doctoral candidates are expected to do their thesis work in connection with ongoing research programs in their own countries. Re-entry grants for those returning home from doctoral training (whether supported by TDR or not) are now available.

• Fellowships are now available for a limited number of post-doctoral fellows who want to obtain practical hands-on field experience.

• Program-based grants are a new approach for support of institutions, often involving integration of laboratory-based research with clinical and field studies, and with linkages to other research groups.

• Linkages with strong research groups in industrialized countries have been found to facilitate greatly the transfer of skills to institutions in developing countries. TDR has joined with the Rockefeller Foundation to support a number of such research and training linkages.

• FIELDLINCS (Field Linkages for Intervention and Control Studies) is a new initiative to strengthen multidisciplinary field research, especially for trials of new intervention tools.

• Career development grants are another new form of support that will be available to a limited number of outstanding young investigators for periods of up to five years, to overcome the many barriers that divert potential researchers to other endeavors.

Although TDR has made a substantial effort to help establish post-graduate epidemiological capacity in a number of institutions, it has become clear that the development of such training capabilities is a very long-term and very large effort, requiring strengths in clinical, laboratory and social sciences as well as public health. The main role for TDR in the next several years will be to provide support for ongoing field research and encourage the use of these field research areas for training purposes. In addition, other efforts to strengthen epidemiological and field research training such as those of INCLEN and the Field Epidemiological Training Program should be encouraged and promoted.

The greatest need for TDR in the next decade is the establishment of field trial capabilities. In addition, an area of complementary research of increasing importance is that of health systems research. To justify the introduction of any new product or strategy, decisions should be based on the relative effectiveness per unit of expenditure. Developing these planning and management capabilities extends well beyond TDR's mandate, but unless the endemic countries establish these capabilities, large investments in basic and applied research and the development of new tools and products will be largely wasted.

---

pate in such research. The elements needed for successful contributions to global health research are highly qualified scientists in the relevant disciplines, adequate research support, and good linkages to a network of peers worldwide. Now and in the future, more and more developing countries are and will be in a position to contribute to global health research.

National Commitment

Building capacity for research in developing countries—for both country-specific research and global re-

Box 8.5 A regional individual awards program in the Middle East

The Middle East Awards Program in Population and Development (MEAwards) was established in 1978 and has been supported by the Ford Foundation, IDRC, and the Population Council. MEAwards is a regional program that helps develop individual research capacity by funding research, fellowships, study groups, and training workshops in population, reproductive health, and child survival. The program is administered by a secretariat based at the regional offices of the Population Council in Cairo.

Awards, which are made by a committee of Arab and Turkish social scientists, range from $5,000 to $35,000 for work carried out mainly in the region. Awards are contingent upon the quality of the submitted proposals; if necessary, technical assistance is provided to researchers at the preparatory stage when the MEAwards staff or committee see promise in an application. Administrative and technical assistance by the program comprise 26 percent of the total budget, which averages about $350,000 annually.

In its first decade, MEAwards provided 59 research grants, funded 65 publications, and awarded 42 fellowships. In 1987, three working groups were established, forming regional networks of scientists concerned with child survival and development, women's reproductive health, and women's resources and management of health in the household.

search—requires strong commitment by political, financial, and health leaders, backed by an informed and supportive public. Such commitment is necessary to mobilize national support to build career structures, incentives, and funding for creating and sustaining research capacity. The Third World Academy of Sciences has proposed a target of 2 percent of GNP as a necessary minimum investment to develop a nation's science and technology capabilities. Health might expect to receive at least 10 percent of such science and technology investments. External aid can assist in, but cannot substitute for, this national commitment (Box 8.1, page 72).

International Response

Because external aid constitutes a significant portion of health research funding, and because donor funds are often more flexible than national funds, investment decisions by funding agencies are critical to building and sustaining research capacity in developing countries. Our review of donor activities has shown that the overall efforts of donors are inadequate in several respects. Overall budgetary commitments to capacity building are small, totaling less than $50 million annually, or less than 5 percent of the total funds invested in health research on developing-country health problems.[2] Only a few small donors—mainly foundations—give priority to capacity building. Particularly disappointing is the low priority accorded to capacity building by bilateral aid agencies and development banks. The large project and program aid flows often make use of research capacity built by others but do not direct a share of their own investments toward capacity building in developing countries. There are, moreover, insufficient investments being made in longer-term advanced training. Rather, the preference appears to be for brief in-country or regional training. While clearly valuable and more affordable, these short-term exchanges cannot substitute for longer-term formal training.

To their credit, the private foundations have consistently pursued capacity building as a principal component of their program strategies. This has been true of older foundations, such as the Rockefeller, Ford, and Kellogg foundations, the Carnegie Corporation, and the Wellcome Trust; newer foundations have also become increasingly engaged, such as the Aga Khan and Sasakawa foundations and the Pew Charitable Trusts (Box 8.2, page 73). Indeed, the Ford Foundation noted in its annual report that "In all fields, the principal approach is to develop local competence, both among individuals and institutions, and help apply it to the solution of development problems."[3] Capacity building has also been a hallmark of programs by IDRC in Canada

and SAREC in Sweden (Box 8.3, page 73).

In general, capacity building has not been a high priority for most multilateral agencies. Important leadership in research capacity building has been shown by the HRP and TDR programs. HRP devotes a substantial portion of its annual $20 million budget to capacity building. In its first decade, TDR invested over $40 million in capacity building and recently announced plans

---

Box 8.6 Building nutritional research capacity: INCAP and UNU

In 1946 representatives of the ministries of health from the six countries of Central America and Panama met to plan the Institute of Nutrition of Central America and Panama (INCAP). The institute they created had three objectives: to determine the nutritional problems of the region; to find practical solutions through research; and to assist member countries in the application of solutions through advisory services, education, and training.

Several organizational provisions helped ensure that INCAP was able to maintain its course in addressing its mandate. The Governing Council was created as an oversight mechanism, representing the ministers of health from the six countries. Additionally, an administrative relationship was established between the Pan American Health Organization and INCAP.

Internal policy provisions helped to ensure the quality and appropriateness of research, as well as to promote indigenous research capacity. A scientific advisory committee met annually to review and advise on all activities; external support for research was targeted for INCAP-designed projects that met the perceived needs of member countries; every project proposal was submitted for internal technical review as well as to the Governing Council for approval. Moreover, initial staff members were all Central Americans, and professional interaction with students and researchers at Central American universities and medical schools was actively encouraged.

Patterned after the experience in building INCAP, the United Nations University (UNU) program for institution building in nutrition focused on the advanced training of key personnel in developing-country institutions capable of making important contributions to research, training, and policy advice in food and nutrition. Institutions for assistance were selected by site visit and discussion of staff development needs. Fellowships were awarded only on the basis of personal interview and assurance from the institution that those selected would be given the opportunity to make use of the additional training.

Most were sent to UNU-associated institutions that agreed to provide training specially adapted to the needs of the fellow and the home institution. As often as possible, fellows were sent to associated institutions such as INCAP that are located in developing countries. More than 500 fellows have been supported since 1986.

to integrate this component of its program more closely with its research activities and focus more strongly on epidemiological and field research capacities (Box 8.4, page 74). Capacity building is not a primary objective of the CDD program, and the generously funded GPA has yet to articulate a capacity-building strategy, in spite of the fact that both programs (and others such as EPI) make heavy demands on the limited personnel available in developing countries to carry out epidemiological, socioeconomic, and anthropological studies and clinical field trials. UNDP and the World Bank have until recently supported capacity building primarily through their support of HRP and TDR; both agencies are now considering direct investment in capacity building in sub-Saharan Africa. UNICEF also has recently begun a capacity-building program for child survival and devel-

opment in Africa. UNFPA has been a major source of support for capacity building in the fields of national statistics and demography throughout the developing world.

In Chapter 7 it was noted that the donor agencies with the greatest untapped potential for health research promotion are the bilateral assistance agencies. The same observation can be made about their contribution to research capacity building. Because of their dominant focus on project and program aid, research capacity building, like research, currently receives low priority. In part, the problem is the limited availability of staff and their time. More serious constraints are those posed by official mandates and political expectations, which are often oriented to short-term results. Within USAID, for example, capacity building is no longer accorded

Table 8.1 Selected international programs to support research and capacity building in epidemiology, health policy, and management

PROGRAM	FOCUS	TARGET	APPROACHES TO TRAINING	YEAR ESTABLISHED	FELLOWS OR TRAINEES
WHO-sponsored					
HSR[a]	Health and health systems	Trainers, managers, policy makers	Workshops, consultative meetings, courses	1982	140 total
HE[b]	Health economics	Program managers, policy makers	Short courses, workshops	—	—
HRP[c]	Fertility regulation, infertility	Scientists, policymakers	Fellowships, workshops, courses	1971–72	—
TDR[c]	Tropical diseases	Scientists, policymakers	Fellowships, workshops, courses	1974	—
Other Sponsors					
COEIHS[d]	Human resource development for health care	Educators, policymakers	Community-based curricula focused on priority health problems	1979	10–15 total annually
IHPP[e]	Health policy	Scientists, policymakers	Institutional support, fellowships	1986	15–20 total
INCLEN[f]	Clinical epi., biostat, hlth econ; social sciences	Clinical faculty	Fellowships and institutional support	1981	235 total
NEB[g]	Epi. and health policy	Scientists, policymakers	—	1985	—
CEN[h]	Epi. and health management	Program managers, policymakers,	Short courses backed by overseas support	1986	90 projected
FETP[i]	Public health applications of epi.	Public health officers	Short courses; in-service training, backed by CDC	1980	110 graduates, 85 in training

a. Programme on Health Systems Research and Development
b. Health Economics
c. Epidemiology and socioeconomic elements of HRP and TDR
d. Network of Community-Oriented Educational Institutions for Health Sciences
e. International Health Policy Program

f. International Clinical Epidemiology Network
g. National Epidemiology Boards
h. Community Epidemiology and Health Management Network
i. Field Epidemiology Training Program of the United States Centers for Disease Control

the priority it had some decades ago. The recent USAID concern over the "sustainability" of child survival action efforts may pave the way for a resurgence of attention to capacity building.

New Strategies

Given the constraints on research institutions, the magnitude of the resources required and the limited resources available, what are the most effective strategies for capacity building?

Institutional strengthening

Research capacity building requires capable management and stable support of institutions over an extended period, usually 10 to 15 years. Too little attention is given to the quality of research management, and short-term or intermittent funding leads to waste and in-

PRINCIPAL GEOGRAPHIC FOCUS	PRIMARY SPONSORS
Africa, Asia, Latin America	Dutch govt., DANIDA
Africa, Asia, South America	USAID, DANIDA
China, Latin America, Sub-Saharan Africa	UNDP, UNFPA, World Bank, WHO
—	UNDP, World Bank, WHO
Global	WHO, universities, several foundations
Southeast Asia, Sub-Saharan Africa	Pew and Carnegie Foundations
Africa, Asia, Latin America, India	Rockefeller Foundation
Thailand, Mexico, Cameroon	Rockefeller Foundation
India, Indonesia	Ford Foundation
Americas, W. Pacific, E. Mediterranean, S.E. Asia	National budgets, CDC, WHO, USAID

NOTE: This table is intended only to display several examples; it is not a complete listing of programs in this field.

Source: Compiled from recent reports and personal communications with each of the programs listed.

efficiency. In some situations donors provide too much money for a short period, failing to recognize that, given limited absorptive capacity, an institution would be better served by smaller grants over a longer period. Some agencies have supported specific institutions for long periods, but, from the developing-country perspective, the need for renewals every two or three years creates a climate of uncertainty that leads to short-term planning. Much better results would be obtained from an initial long-term commitment to an institution by a donor agency subject only to achieving reasonable milestones and to the normal legal caveats of the agency. Recognizing the wide differences among institutions and national circumstances, donor agencies can enhance the impact of their investments by adapting their processes to local needs, avoiding bureaucratic rigidity, and not restricting their support to narrow subject areas.

Professional and career development

Appropriate professional training, support, and career incentives are key factors in attracting outstanding young professionals and nurturing their growth and development (Box 8.5, page 74). Investments can support professional training by channeling funds through selected institutions, or via an open process intended to give professionals greater skills, after which institutions would be expected to compete for talent. Training can be free-standing or integrated with specific research activities. Particularly useful for advanced training is the "sandwich" model, in which researchers train abroad for advanced skills, return to developing countries for a substantial period of fieldwork, and complete their training abroad with a period of analysis and writing. Such an approach leads to competence development while remaining relevant to developing-country issues.

Equally important are strategies to overcome the difficulties for researchers created by too few numbers—or lack of a "critical mass"—and intellectual isolation. Conferences, workshops, access to literature, and sabbatical time abroad are all useful. In this regard, the strategic focus should be on the professional in his or her home country, rather than on an external program. These complementary short-term activities can become excessively concentrated on a few outstanding people who are overextended, while more junior investigators who would benefit most may not be given the opportunity to participate. National and regional programs, with strong capacity-building components, tend to be more effective for attracting and building competence in junior researchers (Box 8.6, page 75).

Networking

Networking is a useful mechanism to provide in-

Box 8.7 Regional networking: the SEAMEO-TROPMED model

The Southeast Asian Ministers of Education Organization (SEAMEO), an intergovernmental group of eight member states, established its Tropical Medicine and Public Health Project (TROPMED) in 1967 to improve health in Southeast Asia. The project offers postgraduate training in tropical medicine and public health and supports research in tropical diseases, all on a cooperative regional basis.

With a secretariat based in Bangkok, TROPMED works chiefly through four national centers for training and research in Indonesia, Malaysia, the Philippines, and Thailand. Each center is a fully equipped school with laboratories, classrooms, and in some cases, hospital beds. To avoid duplication, each center has an agreed-upon area of specialization. Thus, TROPMED can provide strong training in complementary areas without diluting the focus of participating centers. Each center grants postgraduate degrees and sponsors research in subjects ranging from applied nutrition to health economics to medical microbiology.

Operations and staffing of TROPMED's national centers are paid for by their host countries, while support of the secretariat is jointly shared by the four countries. Special funds for fellowships, research grants, faculty exchanges, seminars, and meetings come from various donor groups, including SEAMEO member countries and foreign agencies.

TROPMED trains about 150 Asian scientists yearly. Thousands of professionals, 80 percent of them from Southeast Asia, have attended TROPMED seminars and conferences. The project publishes a quarterly medical journal as well as proceedings of its seminars and conferences.

ternational support and communication for scientists while at the same time strengthening national research capacity. The network can achieve depth and diversity of research capability that would not be possible in individual institutions. The network may also buffer a national institution during a period of political instability. The chief disadvantages are the time and effort necessary to make a multicenter program operate well. HRP and TDR are examples of successful international networks; a successful regional network is the SEAMEO/-TROPMED program in Southeast Asia (Box 8.7). Regional associations, such as SAARC, SADCC, and the Commonwealth Secretariat, are good organizational bases for the creation of networks. Other international arrangements include various exchanges among developing-country institutions as well as twinning arrangements between developing-country and industrialized-country institutions.

The Special Needs of Country-Specific Health Research

The disciplines and institutional structures critical to country-specific health research are weak in nearly all countries and particularly so in the developing countries that most need this type of research. In addition to capacity building at the national level, international support and public recognition for this neglected field are required.

Currently several international programs, some sponsored by WHO and some by other organizations, are seeking to build capacity in developing countries for country-specific health research; they include WHO's Health Systems Research (HSR) and Health Economics programs, the social science and field research components of HRP and TDR, INCLEN, IHPP, and others (Table 8.1, pages 76–77). These programs, though most-

Box 8.8 Human and institutional development in Africa

One impediment to national development in Africa has been the relative lack of human and institutional capacity for designing, managing, and evaluating interventions at the community level. In response to this gap, several international initiatives are either underway or under active planning.

The **International Child Development Centre** (ICDC), a new UNICEF facility established in Florence through the support of the government of Italy, has created a Special Programme on National Capacity Building for Child Survival and Development in Africa. Working with African universities, governments, nongovernmental organizations, and community groups, the program seeks to foster a self-sustaining learning process within African countries aimed toward the solution of local problems related to the changing needs of children. In addition to pro-

moting national initiatives, the program is facilitating linkages at the regional and international levels by "twinning" and "networking" developing-country institutions with outstanding learning centers in other parts of the world.

Another international initiative focused on support for capacity building in sub-Saharan Africa is being developed by the **World Bank**. Following a recent review of development policies and strategies in Africa, the Bank has decided to place new emphasis on building and sustaining human and organizational capabilities for policy analysis and management in Africa. One possible follow-up action would be the formulation of a special capacity-building fund for supporting, with increased resources, the development of long-term capabilities in the region; health would be one of the fields supported by this initiative.

ly small and recently established, offer much promise of assisting the growth of individual and institutional competence in health-systems research, health economics, epidemiology, policy analysis, and other elements that are urgently needed for country-specific health research. These programs should be strengthened and their efforts coordinated at the country level to facilitate an integrated rather than separate approach to building country-specific research capability in developing countries.

Efforts toward integration at the national level should be reinforced by an annual international meeting of scientists, health and development leaders, and donor representatives interested in country-specific health research, sponsored by development agencies and foundations, to promote the exchange of information on research results and methods and to mobilize financial and technical assistance.

To provide a career incentive and peer and public recognition for scientists working in country-specific health research, it would be desirable to establish international awards to be presented at the annual meeting to three to five young leaders in the field for distinguished contributions to country-specific research.

The Special Needs of Sub-Saharan Africa

Sub-Saharan Africa deserves special consideration for health research capacity building because health problems have been aggravated by economic, environmental, and political difficulties and national resources to respond are severely limited. The region clearly needs accelerated and intensive efforts both by national governments and by the international donor community. The extensive use of highly paid foreign technical advisors by many development agencies should be reexamined in favor of more cost-effective direct investments in African professionals and institutions. Fresh strategies should be pursued. UNDP and the World Bank are now establishing broad capacity-strengthening programs in African countries, and health research capacity would be included as one objective. UNICEF, as mentioned, has initiated a program to strengthen capacity in government, universities, and nongovernmental agencies for child survival and development in Africa over the next five years (Box 8.8). Innovative schemes, such as a special career development program for African scientists, should be considered.

Conclusions

1. Building and sustaining research capacity within developing countries is an essential and effective means of accelerating research contributions to health and development. Nurturing individual scientific competence and leadership, strengthening institutions, establishing strong linkages between research and action agencies, and reinforcing national institutions through international networks are all important elements of capacity building.

2. Capacity building for country-specific health research should be given top priority by every country because of its importance to policy and management decisions for the health sector. It is equally important to create demand for research results among those responsible for health policy and management through effective arrangements for communication and shared priority setting for research.

3. National commitment is indispensable to secure the resources and to create a positive environment for research capacity building.

4. Bilateral and multilateral agencies and development banks should reduce their dependence on expatriate consultants and increase their investment in research capacity in developing countries. Special attention should be given to sub-Saharan African countries.

5. Capacity building requires sustained support over an extended period. External agencies can assist more effectively by committing at the outset support for 10 to 15 years subject only to demonstrating achievement in relation to agreed-upon milestones and normal agency legal and reporting requirements.

Part Three

An Agenda for Action

CHAPTER 9

An Agenda for Action

Our study has led us to a broad vision of health research for development—of how health and development are mutually interdependent and how health research can help accelerate health improvements in developing countries. That vision includes four interrelated elements.

1. Health and development

The powerful linkages between health and development must be recognized and acted upon. Health investments should be accorded high priority by development planners and finance agencies, both in developing countries and in the international community. Health, like education, is often perceived as a "soft" consumption sector which will only follow advances in "harder" sectors like industry and agriculture. The converse, we argue, is equally true. Investing wisely in health will build human capital, enabling people on a more equitable basis to contribute to and gain from economic productivity. Unlike investments in factories and roads, investments in health can generate returns that do not depreciate and that can bring significant social benefits for a lifetime and into the next generation.

2. Research: the essential basis for action and equity

The key role of research in improving health, especially the health of disadvantaged groups, must be recognized by developing-country governments and international development agencies. Health research is a vital investment in the future. The seeds of research that are sown today will yield a wealth of effective action tomorrow. Health research serves two powerful purposes:

First, a core amount of research is essential in every country to determine its particular health problems, to analyze different measures for dealing with them, and to help in the choice of appropriate actions that will achieve the greatest health improvement with limited resources. Country-specific research is needed not only to serve the national government, but also to enable communities, households, and individuals to take more appropriate and effective health action. These research tasks are continuously evolving and require the development of health information and research capacity to guide decision-makers in the context of rapid economic, social, demographic, and environmental change. With the re-

> *As one species, we share a common vulnerability. . . . No matter how selfish our motives, we can no longer be indifferent to the suffering of others. The microbe that felled one child in a distant continent yesterday can reach yours today and seed a global pandemic tomorrow. "'Never send to know for whom the bell tolls; it tolls for thee."*
>
> **Joshua Lederberg**
> *President,*
> *Rockefeller University*

sults of country-specific research, leaders not only can make well-informed decisions about allocating the country's own resources but can also ensure that assistance from the international community is applied in a manner that reinforces national health purposes and plans.

Second, health research develops new knowledge and technologies to cope with major unsolved health problems worldwide. For many key health problems, the need for new tools is urgent. Global research collaboration, bringing together scientists from industrialized and developing countries, is urgently needed to find better and lower-cost means for dealing with many health problems for which existing knowledge does not provide solutions at affordable costs.

3. *Building developing-country research capacity*

Stronger research capabilities are needed within developing countries to empower them to advance the health status of their own people, particularly low-income groups, and to contribute to health progress worldwide.

Overcoming the imposing obstacles to improving health in the Third World requires that the affected countries exercise initiative and leadership to make the most of the limited resources they have to spend on health, and to seek from elsewhere additional knowledge and resources to match their own priorities. As the foundation for their initiative and leadership, scientific research capacity is vital. Currently, there is heavy reliance on scientists in industrialized countries for making research advances on health problems of developing countries. But the present imbalance is a transient historical phase, with scientists in some developing countries already making world-class contributions. In many other Third World countries, scientists are growing in number, competence, and experience. In the future, the involvement of industrialized-country scientists should be sustained and increased, but there should be disproportionately larger increases in the quantity and quality of developing-country researchers and institutions.

4. *International health interdependence*

In health as in other fields, the world is becoming a global village. Worldwide health threats are increasing: AIDS, substance abuse, environmental hazards. There are, correspondingly, common needs for improved management of shared diseases, development of drugs and devices, international standards for training personnel, and innovations in health care. To an increasing degree industrialized and developing countries share the same health problems; the differences are in the way they respond, the availability of resources, and the strength of their institutions. There are compelling reasons for common action: self-interest for self-protection, opportunities to learn from each other's experiences, and humanitarian desires to reduce gross inequities.

We thus argue for a strengthening of an international health research system—a system in which developing-country researchers will play critical roles. We see this system yielding very large benefits in reducing global health inequities and in contributing to the solution of health problems worldwide.

Major Findings

Our assessment of worldwide health research for development has identified the major challenges, the principal actors, the many constraints faced, and the gaps and weaknesses that need attention. These findings show that:

• The worldwide flow of resources supporting research on health problems of developing countries is very limited, and its application leaves large gaps. Greater amounts and more efficient application of resources are needed to support a major expansion and improvement of research activities and capacity within developing countries.

• The enormous diversity of health circumstances speaks to the importance of priority setting at the national and international levels. Several major health problems are receiving attention; others appear relatively neglected. Major gaps exist with regard to information, monitoring, and assessment of the evolving health picture. Greater coherence of research responses to high-priority problems at the national and international levels is needed.

• Developing-country scientists and institutions are pursuing a wide range of research activities, but greater productivity will require overcoming serious constraints—professional, institutional, and environmental. National commitment and international reinforcement for health research, specific actions to tackle constraints, and capacity building and maintenance within developing countries will all be necessary.

• Appropriate contributions from industrialized countries should be expanded, focusing on advanced training, research, technical interaction, and participation in international partnership arrangements. Rather than a system of new independent international centers, the major emphasis should be given to strengthening national centers and achieving "critical mass" and shared objectives through international networks of national centers.

• The number and type of international research promotion programs are growing. These constitute the beginnings of a worldwide health research system. Joint efforts by United Nations agencies are noteworthy, and privately sponsored efforts have been productive. Stronger overall coherence is needed to reduce the fragmentation and competition induced by multiple, narrowly focused research initiatives.

• Far too little attention is being given to the critical importance of building and sustaining individual and institutional health research capacity within developing countries. To remedy this problem, leadership and commitment by national governments as well as longer-term support by international agencies will be necessary.

An Action Agenda

To meet these challenges, we propose an agenda for action that has four components:
• essential national health research in all countries, but especially in developing countries;
• international partnerships to facilitate collaboration of scientists from all countries in global health challenges;
• building and sustaining in both developing and industrialized countries individual and institutional research capacity concerned with Third World health problems; and
• improved international arrangements (international reinforcement and financing) for monitoring, assessment, and promotion of research on health problems of developing countries.

Essential national health research
To understand its own problems, to enhance the impact of limited resources, to improve health policy and management, to foster innovation and experimentation, and to provide the foundation for a stronger developing-country voice in setting international priorities, the establishment and strengthening of an appropriate health research base in each developing country, no matter how poor, is essential. This Commission has named such a base *essential national health research.* ENHR is important to national governments, nongovernmental agencies, regional and district health service managers, health workers, communities, families, and individuals. Exactly what mix of research is essential must be defined by each country, but it will contain some measure of two basic components, country-specific health research and global health research.

The work most seriously neglected at present is country-specific research that can inform decision-making on health action. This kind of research is aimed at defining the health situation (e.g., the prevalence of AIDS, tuberculosis, and immunizable diseases), shaping health policy (e.g., the financing of health services, the

rational use of therapeutic drugs), and improving program operations (e.g., management information systems). The challenges in conducting country-specific research are daunting because it involves governmental and nongovernmental groups, often must transcend disciplinary boundaries, deals with professionally and politically sensitive problems, and requires researchers to interact with users of the results of research in governmental and nongovernmental agencies. Constraints at present to the promotion and use of country-specific research include low appreciation and weak demand among policymakers, poor public understanding, conflicting priorities of funding agencies, and deeply ingrained disciplinary and professional attitudes that hamper its acceptance.

Some developing countries, nevertheless, have launched efforts in country-specific research, although most of these are recent and still fragile. Several international programs are making useful contributions, among them the WHO programs in health economics, health systems research, and district management, as well as portions of the research and training programs in tropical diseases and human reproduction; UNICEF's evaluation activities and sentinel site surveys; and foundation-sponsored research initiatives in clinical and community epidemiology, management, and health policy. These programs, however, are small and narrowly focused in relation to the broad overall need for the systematic pursuit of country-specific research in all countries.

A second aspect of ENHR is research in each developing country on global health problems that affect its population. Many aspects of global health research must be carried out in the field conditions of developing countries, such as trials of new vaccines for tropical diseases and tests of nutritional supplements such as vitamin A. Beyond this, laboratory-based biomedical research on tropical diseases is increasingly being done in Third World institutions, of which Mahidol University in Bangkok and the Oswaldo Cruz Foundation in Rio de Janeiro are but two leading examples. Every country must decide what it can contribute to the international effort to master the world's unsolved health problems. Together, developing countries have the largest stake in the outcome and can mobilize steadily larger and more sophisticated research communities.

We recommend that each country develop a strong national plan to conduct research on both country-specific and global health problems—a plan that is feasible, economical, and coherent and that involves all relevant groups. Implementing such a plan will require building and maintaining research capacity within developing countries and sustained reinforcement from the international community. A critical mass of health researchers is needed in every country, nurtured by improved career paths, including incentives and rewards. The research capacity should be closely linked to the policymakers, managers, and other users of the results of research. Government support is essential. We recommend that all governments commit 2 percent of their health budgets for ENHR.

International partnerships

Tackling major global health problems requires that scientific and financial resources be directed at key problems. The aim should be to strengthen and enlarge the international system for research to develop new knowledge and tools. Tackling country-specific health problems also calls for international partnerships to share methods and results and to join in collaborative research. In these processes, greater voice and participation should be accorded to developing-country groups; and industrialized-country groups have much to gain as well as to contribute.

A pluralistic worldwide health research system is already emerging, and some important health problems, such as the tropical diseases, human reproduction, diarrhea, and AIDS, are receiving focused international attention. Other problems, however—some equally significant—are badly neglected, among them acute respiratory disease, tuberculosis, sexually transmitted diseases, chronic diseases and injuries, mental illness, and behavioral health problems.

Chronic and degenerative diseases are already evident as an increasingly important component of the disease burden of developing countries. Innovative preventive and therapeutic strategies beyond the technologies currently available will be required to meet the challenge of these diseases at affordable costs. Studies of risk factors predisposing people to chronic and degenerative diseases assume special significance because they hold out the possibility that the high prevalence in industrialized countries could be avoided in developing countries. New health threats are also emerging, such as substance abuse (drugs, alcohol, and tobacco), occupational hazards, and environmental threats.

We recommend that steadily increasing attention and funds be given to the building of international partnerships to speed up the conduct of research and the widespread dissemination of results. In recognition of increasing worldwide health interdependence, greater public awareness of health challenges and stronger policy support for research on neglected problems are needed. There is need for systematic review of existing research programs to ensure appropriate continuing support and for a mechanism to promote research on important neglected problems.

Building and sustaining research capacity in developing countries

One of the most cost-effective means to support both ENHR and international partnerships is to build and sustain research capacity in developing countries.

Research capacity in developing countries is diverse. Some extremely capable researchers and institutions are undertaking high-quality research, often leading international advances. Capacity in most developing countries, however, is small and inadequately supported. Country-specific health research is especially weak and is rarely a priority of medical schools or national research councils. The capacity to contribute to global health research is also weak in all but a handful of developing countries. At present, international support is limited to a narrow range of specific diseases. A major long-term effort is required to rectify these deficiencies.

We recommend that building and sustaining research capacity be integrated as a key objective and powerful instrument for all health and development investments. Primary commitment must come from developing-country governments to accord priority and provide sustained financial support. Strong international reinforcement is also needed. International exchange and interaction can do a great deal to help strengthen the capacity of developing-country researchers and institutions.

Donors and international programs should earmark funds for capacity building. Health projects, both those supported domestically and those with foreign funding, should be used to build new capabilities rather than diverting existing ones from other work. Donor-assisted health projects should commit at least 5 percent of the project budget to research capacity strengthening and research activities.

Capacity building for research has not been a priority with most donor agencies because it is costly and time-consuming and does not seem to produce immediate results. Strategies such as "sandwich" training between home and foreign centers, twinning relationships, and networking all hold promise for faster and more effective returns on investments.

International reinforcement

Recognition, promotion, facilitation, and investment by international agencies and donor groups are needed to advance both ENHR and international partnerships.

For country-specific research, we recommend the establishing or strengthening of networks at the national, regional, and international levels. The networks would serve as a mechanism to assist in-country efforts as well as to perform key international functions including advocacy, education, promotion, and the mobilization of technical and financial resources. International technical programs with research and training capability should be strengthened to provide maximum support at the country level. We recommend that a facilitation unit to strengthen country-specific research be established to help developing countries achieve more efficient and effective capacity building and to coordinate external linkages. The entity should be sponsored and supported by developing countries, United Nations agencies (e.g., WHO, UNICEF, UNDP, the World Bank), bilateral donors, private foundations, and other interested parties, many of which will benefit from having stronger policy and management capability in place at the country level.

For global health research, international arrangements should build upon existing international programs. Except in unusual circumstances we do not recommend new autonomous international research centers. Rather, we recommend the strengthening of national centers in developing countries and interconnecting them in networks to fulfill both national and international roles. International research programs such as HRP and TDR have evolved, for example, a workable structure of governance drawing upon broad-based participation. They have also developed systems of scientific review to perform technical assessment through working groups and steering committees, help decide upon strategic future directions, and help guide the allocation of research resources. These programs perform very well in focusing on problems within their mandates.

There is a need, however, for a mechanism to monitor the progress of research on developing-country health problems and to identify unmet needs. We recommend that an international mechanism be established to carry out regular, systematic reviews of research addressing high-priority health problems. The mechanism should be responsible for monitoring, assessment, convening, and advocacy. It should not be an executing agency. It must have the credibility to attract participation of the relevant parties—developing countries, UN and international agencies, bilateral donors, and the scientific community. It must have sufficient resources to produce information of high quality which is not available from other sources. It should be independent of particular interests—geographical, bureaucratic, or scientific.

Financing research for health and development

The challenge of responding to the health inequities and health research disparities facing developing countries is both to expand the pool of financial and human resources directed at developing-world health problems, and simultaneously to improve the efficiency, effectiveness, and equity impact of existing investments. Expanding the resource pool requires an understanding of the incentive structure that determines the flow of governmental and private sector resources.

How are these resource flows likely to respond to the needs of international health research, and for what reasons? Leaders of developing nations must see political rewards, development gains, and welfare improvements from health research investments. Likewise, public and parliamentary bodies in industrialized countries must see their humanitarian goals and self-interests served by investments in both country-specific and global health research.

The potential for change from the private sector, comprising foundations and industry, is modest. Total foundation investments are unlikely to grow substantially, except from foundations in Japan; however, foundation preference for research investments is high and should be further encouraged. Industry, on the other hand, lacks incentives to develop products for economically weak markets, and this limits pharmaceutical companies' interest in research on health problems of developing countries. Innovative responses oriented toward industry's profit motivations and social obligations are required to encourage companies to play a larger role in international health research.

We believe that future expansion of international health research capacity, which if used well can save large sums in health action programs, is likely to occur largely in the developing world. The efficiency, effectiveness, and equity impact of existing health research resources depend not only upon the amount of available funds, but also upon the capacity of developing countries to absorb those funds and use them well. The outcome also depends upon the quality and effectiveness of international research promotion mechanisms that support research on health problems of developing countries.

Summary of Specific Recommendations

Essential National Health Research

1. We find that essential national health research (ENHR) is a critical tool for equitable health and development and therefore recommend that each developing country, taking account of its own circumstances, make careful plans for and carry out sustained, long-term programs for building research capacity and conducting ENHR.

2. In making plans, each developing country should set its goals in terms of the two principal objectives of ENHR: (a) to identify country-specific health problems and design and evaluate action programs for dealing with them, and (b) to join in the international effort to find new knowledge, methods, and technologies for addressing global health problems that are of high priority for the country in question. These objectives provide a basis for realistic planning for health research facilities that will be aimed at the highest-priority health problems and consistent with what can be afforded over time. At present the most urgent need in virtually every country is for a rapid enlargement of capacity for country-specific health research.

3. To build research capacity for ENHR, each developing country will need:
  • to invest in long-term development of the research capacity of individuals and institutions, especially in neglected fields such as epidemiology, the social and policy sciences, and management research;
  • to set national priorities for research, for using both domestic and external resources;
  • to accord professional recognition of good research and build career paths to attract and retain able researchers;
  • to develop reliable and continuing links between researchers and research users; and

  • to invest at least 2 per cent of national health expenditures in ENHR.

International Partnerships

1. We find that the major health problems of humanity can be addressed most effectively through the cooperative efforts of scientists around the world, and we therefore recommend that developing and industrialized countries and international agencies promote the steady growth of collaborative international research networks as the principal means for mobilizing scientific talent to attack common problems.

2. Some important health problems are being addressed by internationally organized research programs, but other problems are comparatively neglected. The priorities for research will change over time. At present we recommend:
  • continuing and expanded support for two successful existing programs, TDR and HRP;
  • continuing and expanded support for two diarrheal disease programs, CDD and ICDDR,B;
  • rapid expansion of research on acute respiratory infections, with special emphasis on simple and effective treatment;
  • establishment of a research and action program on improved methods for case detection, ambulatory treatment, and prevention of tuberculosis;
  • research in support of national programs to eradicate micronutrient deficiencies, especially of vitamin A, iron, and iodine;
  • collaborative international research to identify modifiable factors to avert the high risk of diabetes, coronary heart disease, and hypertension associated with the health transition; and
  • design and assessment of behavioral interventions to reduce injuries, sexually transmitted diseases,

and the growing threat of substance abuse;

• significant expansion of international collaborative research on mental health problems, emphasizing methods to diagnose and deal with the most prevalent and treatable conditions; and

• establishment of sustained international research networks in the most important areas of environmental and occupational health.

3. An international support system is needed to help developing countries strengthen country-specific health research capacity and action. We recommend that:

• the several international programs—HSR, Health Economics, INCLEN, and IHPP among others—that deal with selected aspects of country-specific health research be sustained and strengthened and coordinate their efforts at country level;

• a facilitation unit to strengthen country-specific research be established to help developing countries achieve more efficient and effective national capacity building and to coordinate external linkages; the entity should be sponsored and supported by developing countries, United Nations agencies, bilateral donors, foundations, and other interested parties;

• an annual meeting of scientists, health leaders, and donor representatives interested in country-specific health research be sponsored by developing countries, development agencies, and foundations to promote information exchange about research results and methods and to mobilize financial and technical assistance;

• international awards for distinguished contributions to country-specific health research be established and presented each year at the annual country-specific health research meeting to three to five young leaders in this field of research.

4. Industrialized-country health research and training institutions are a major resource for addressing health problems of developing countries. We recommend that industrialized countries:

• provide career opportunities for young scientists to become engaged in research on health problems of developing countries;

• promote the strengthening of schools of public health, tropical disease institutes, medical schools, and development studies groups—all of these to pursue advanced research, conduct training of industrialized-country and developing-country scientists, and participate in international networks;

• commit a larger share of the budgets of health research funding agencies to support research focused on health problems of developing countries.

5. We recommend that WHO, UNDP, the development banks, and other agencies strengthen existing international research-promotion programs and augment them where appropriate, increase their own investments in health research and research capacity strengthening, and reinvigorate research review bodies such as the Advisory Committees on Health Research in WHO headquarters and the regional offices.

Mobilizing Research Funding

1. The proposed expansion of research on health problems of developing countries will require substantial increases in funding. We recommend, therefore, that developing countries, bilateral and multilateral development agencies, industrialized-country research agencies, foundations, NGOs, and the pharmaceutical industry all raise funding levels for health research. Specifically:

• developing countries should invest at least 2 percent of national health expenditures in research and research capacity strengthening, and

• at least 5 percent of project and program aid for the health sector from development aid agencies should be earmarked for research and research capacity strengthening.

2. The quality of research and research strengthening efforts, as well as their quantity, needs improvement. Specifically:

• much longer time horizons should be used for research capacity building than has been customary in the past;

• innovative financing strategies such as debt-for-health-research swaps, funding pools, and funding intermediaries should be explored; and

• foundations and special research agencies such as IDRC and SAREC should continue their pioneering roles in addressing new needs in innovative ways and in mobilizing broader support for major research programs.

Forum for Review and Advocacy

We recommend the establishment of an international mechanism to monitor progress in health research and, when needed, to promote financial and technical support for research on health problems of the developing world. The mechanism should be sufficiently independent to be objective in its recommendations, and therefore its mandate should not be to operate research programs but to promote action by others.

NOTES

Chapter 1

1. We follow the WHO definition of health as not only the absence of disease but also a complete state of well-being. We also define primary health care in accord with the Declaration of Alma-Ata 1978: "Primary health care is essential health care based on practical, scientifically sound and socially acceptable methods and technology made universally accessible to individuals and families in the community through their full participation and at a cost that the community and country can afford to maintain at every stage of their development in the spirit of self-reliance and self-determination. It forms an integral part both of the country's health system, of which it is the central function and main focus, and of the overall social and economic development of the community. It is the first level of contact of individuals, the family and community with the national health system bringing health care as close as possible to where people live and work, and constitutes the first element of a continuing health care process."

2. Data on trends in health progress around the world, as partially described in this chapter, are incomplete and of insufficient quality to be precise regarding stagnation or reversal of health conditions in diverse countries around the world. There is ample evidence, however, that health status has stagnated or even deteriorated among many specific population groups in the past decade.

3. According to the *World Development Report 1989*, about 750 million persons lived in 1987 in the high-income market-oriented countries that are members of the OECD. A conservative allowance for persons who lived, by world standards, in privileged circumstances in other countries would be 200–300 million persons. At the other extreme, the *Report* showed that at least 1.6 billion persons reside in countries that have infant mortality levels equal to or above 80 per 1,000 live births and life expectancies around 55 years.

4. We have followed the United Nations classification of developing and industrialized countries. This classification obviously over-simplifies great diversity among countries and is imperfect because many developing countries are rapidly industrializing and many industrialized countries have population groups with health indicators similar to those prevailing in developing countries.

5. Adult mortality data reflect preliminary results of a World Bank study; see Murray 1990. For additional information on this point, see McCord and Freeman 1990.

6. The decline of the historically important infectious and parasitic diseases does not mean that infectious disease in general has been conquered, even in the industrial countries. New conditions create possibilities for the resurgence of old diseases and the emergence of new ones. The resurgence of tuberculosis and malaria, the outbreaks of Legionnaire's disease, Lyme disease, Congo-Crimean Hemorrhagic Fever, and AIDS attest to the existence of reservoirs of potential pathogens and the versatility of known microorganisms. Some chronic diseases may prove to be associated with slow viruses. Our health depends on a permanent struggle between evolving and adapting pathogens and our invention of methods of prevention and treatment.

7. The importance of chronic and degenerative diseases in developing countries has been underestimated. For example, more cancer deaths occur in developing countries than in industrialized ones although cancer mortality rates per population aggregate are greater in industrialized countries. Moreover, there is growing evidence that social change and social class may influence the risk and severity of these chronic diseases. A recent World Bank study (Briscoe et al. 1989) showed that the incidence of chronic disease was greater among lower-class Brazilians.

8. An economic crisis of a different kind is faced by the health systems of industrialized countries. Escalation of health care costs is a problem in every country. Access to and quality of care, affordability, efficiency, and who pays are all concerns deeply felt and articulated by the general public and the political leadership. The United States leads the world in health expenditures (12 percent of GNP), but 15 percent of its population is without any health insurance, and the health status indicators reveal major disparities among different groups.

9. The definition of development is complex. We view development as not simply economic progress but a process that encompasses social, cultural, and ethical development including the promotion of human rights. In this definition, health and well-being of all citizens is critical because it reflects sustainable and equitable development and because good health is a force that can drive the development process.

Chapter 2

1. The history of science has been one of shifting world centers of knowledge among Babylon, Egypt, China, India, Greece, the Arab world, Europe, and for the last century Europe and North America as a whole. However, we look toward a future polycentric science that draws on a diversity of sources. Non-western medicine is already contributing knowledge of medicinal plants, specific techniques such as acupuncture, and a holistic perspective.

2. Research may be described by the problem studied (tropical disease research) or by the purpose of the research (basic versus applied research). Research can be classified by the methods or sciences used (biological versus social sciences). Research may also be described by the place in which the work is undertaken (clinical versus community research).

Chapter 3

1. Our estimate of potential years of life lost was com-

puted by comparing current estimates of mortality patterns in developing and industrialized countries to an arbitrarily assumed full potential of 85 years for populations. Data used in this estimate are based on UN Population Division current estimates of the ages at which people die in developing and industrialized countries.

2. Estimated worldwide health research expenditures, their sources, and the location of research are all based upon a survey by the Commission secretariat. Our definition of research directed to health problems of developing countries included (1) all health research conducted within developing countries and (2) research conducted in industrialized countries on subjects for which the primary beneficiaries are those in the developing world—mainly research on infectious, parasitic, nutritional, and population problems specific to developing countries.

This definition excludes research conducted in industrialized countries addressing the principal health problems of the industrialized world. Such health problems—e.g., cardiovascular diseases and cancer—are gradually rising in relative importance in developing countries. While research in industrialized countries on these commonly shared problems can benefit citizens of developing countries, the investments were not made with developing-country citizens as intended beneficiaries. Moreover, advances against these commonly shared problems which are developed in industrialized countries are often too technology- and cost-intensive for practical use in developing countries.

Wherever possible, we gathered data for 1986. If an organization's fiscal year did not coincide with the calendar year, an average of adjacent fiscal years or the closest fiscal year was accepted as the estimate for calendar year 1986. All financial figures are expressed in U.S. dollars. All figures cited are actual figures at official exchange rates without adjustment for inflation or purchasing power. For further discussion of the Commission's survey, see Murray et al. 1989 (Commission paper).

3. We estimate that if the "low investor" ODA donors were to adopt "medium investor" levels (0.55 percent) of investment in health research, an extra $55 million would be realized. If the "high investor" level (0.7 percent) were attained by all ODA donors, an additional $104 million would be devoted to health research. Finally, we also estimate that if all donors adopted the ODA standard of 0.7 percent of GNP, even without any change in health research investment percentages, a doubling of health research funding from these donors would result.

Chapter 4

1. Commission estimates, prepared by C.J.L. Murray of the Commission staff, are expressed as confidence intervals in recognition of the imprecision of the available data base.

2. The classification of health problems, referred to in a variety of contexts within the report, is necessarily somewhat arbitrary, with categories often not mutually exclusive. Health problems can be classified according to disease (e.g., schistosomiasis), population group affected (e.g., women of childbearing age), or the type of intervention employed (e.g., immunization). A disease such as measles represents a different classification system from a health problem such as environmental contamination.

3. Unpublished statistics reported in 1989 by Susan Hunter as field notes to the Rockefeller Foundation while she was working as a visiting lecturer at Makerere University, Kampala, Uganda.

4. In this Ghanian work, many assumptions were built into the calculations. In this case, health problems have been defined as disease, and for each disease, its incidence, case fatality, average age of onset, average age at death, average life expectancy, and duration of disability or illness were all estimated in order to assess its impact on years of potential life lost. These estimates were often made on the basis of incomplete data.

5. One of the most active recent debates has been over "selective" versus more "comprehensive" approaches to primary health care. Walsh and Warren (1986) proposed a set of global action priorities based upon a comparison of disease significance and the feasibility and cost of their control. Such technical approaches have several advantages, including underscoring the importance of priority setting, making the assumptions underlying priorities explicit, and attempting to rationalize the allocation of health resources. Critics charge that such a technocratic approach ignores the sociopolitical context of primary health care and oversimplifies enormous diversity in developing countries (Rifkin and Walt 1986). Moreover, classifying health problems as diseases automatically accords higher priority to biomedical technological interventions rather than to broader, more comprehensive health promotion and disease prevention strategies in primary health care.

Chapter 5

1. We asked developing-country respondents to provide two main types of information with respect to their countries: (1) a listing of the principal institutions conducting health research and the number of professional researchers in each, and (2) for each institution, the principal sources of financing and whether the financing originates within the country or outside. Respondents were asked to follow our broad definition of health research, which includes studies of health problems based in the social and management sciences as well as in biomedical and clinical sciences. Respondents were also asked, in the case of researchers who are not full-time, to make rough estimates of the percentage of time spent on research. It is important to note that given our limited budget, no attempt was made to achieve strict comparability among the papers prepared in different countries. Consequently, the results should be interpreted as generally indica-

tive but not precisely comparable.

2. This point is emphasized in the report of the Commission workshop on health research for development, Oswaldo Cruz Foundation, Rio de Janeiro, Brazil, October 11–13 1989.

3. Cabral 1989 (contributed paper).

Chapter 6

1. Despite their obvious importance and major contributions, there have been few systematic studies of research institutions in industrialized countries that focus on health problems of developing countries. Some national studies or disease-focused studies are available from some industrialized countries (see BOSTID/IOM 1987; also Advisory Council for Scientific Research in Development Problems 1984).

2. The citing of specific groups in this section is not intended to slight other equally important groups. Rather, the purpose is to be illustrative and specific in the absence of comprehensive and systematic information on the full range of relevant institutions.

3. This chapter, which addresses the role of industrialized countries, focuses on North-South scientific relationships. There are also very important gains to be achieved in South-South collaboration and in North-North cooperation.

4. The "reverse" learning by which industrialized countries gain from research advances in developing countries is an often neglected aspect of North-South collaboration.

Chapter 7

1. We define research promotion agencies and programs as those bodies that do not undertake research themselves but rather fund, direct, support, and facilitate research undertaken by others. In some ways, these functions in industrialized countries are fulfilled by medical research councils and national academies or national institutes of health.

Chapter 8

1. SAREC defines research capacity as "the ability to independently identify and define research tasks and their relationship to problems and development activities; the ability to select, plan and carry out important research, or to commission or direct such research which cannot successfully be undertaken with domestic technological, financial, and human resources; the ability to assess, sift and adapt research results for domestic application; the ability to offer the country's own research workers an environment which is sufficiently stimulating to counteract migration to technologically advanced countries; the ability to disseminate and apply research results; the ability, in terms of finance and staff, to utilize and participate in the opportunities offered by international research cooperation" (SAREC 1976).

2. Our estimate of financial commitment for capacity building is necessarily uncertain, because few donors report expenditures for capacity building separately. To arrive at this figure, we used conservative assumptions, classifying as capacity-building investments only those expenditures specifically targeted at capacity building purposes (Harkavy and Diescho 1989; Commission paper).

3. Ford Foundation 1987.

BIBLIOGRAPHIC NOTES

Chapter 1

This chapter has benefited from the ideas of many previous commissions, including the Independent Commission on International Development Issues (the Brandt Commission), the Independent Commission on International Humanitarian Issues, the International Commission for the Study of Communication Problems, and the World Commission on Environment and Development (the Brundtland Commission). The section on health and development draws from a large body of work, especially that of Abel-Smith 1978; Abel-Smith and Creese 1989; Alleyne 1989; Behrman 1988; Birdsall 1989; Bradley 1977; Evans 1981; FAO 1984; Gopalan 1989; Halstead et al. 1985; Ingram 1989; the International Fund for Agricultural Development 1983; Lipton and de Kadt 1988; Mosley, Jamison, and Henderson 1990; Ramalingaswami 1988, Rifkin and Walt 1986; UNACC/SCN 1989; and Wilson 1988. Discussions of health and epidemiological transitions as well as population issues derive in part from the published work of Caldwell and Caldwell 1989, Frenk et al. 1989 (contributed paper), Keyfitz 1982, Omran 1971, and Preston 1976.

Data used in this chapter were primarily from the World Bank 1989, the United Nations 1986, UNICEF 1989, the U.S. Department of Health and Human Services (n.d.), and the World Health Organization 1978, 1987[b], and 1988. *Box 1.1 (A decade of primary health care)*, in addition to the chapter materials cited above, is based on the ideas of Chen 1986; Herz and Measham 1987, Caldwell and Caldwell 1989; Evans, Hall, and Warford 1981; Murray 1987; the Task Force for Child Survival 1988; Walsh and Warren 1979; and Halstead, Walsh, and Warren 1985. *Box 1.2 (Health and economic crisis)* derives from work of Albanez et al. 1989, Behrman 1988, Cornia et al. 1987, Tucker 1989, and Pinstrup-Anderson 1987. *Box 1.3 (Rapid population growth)* draws on the work of Keyfitz 1989 and, for data, the UN 1985 and 1988. *Box 1.4 (Environmental risks and health)* is based on material from the Bhopal Working Group 1987, Cairncross 1989 (Commission paper), Huddle et al. 1987, McCracken and Conway 1987, Repetto 1985, Wolman 1980, and the World Resources Institute 1987. *Box 1.5 (Nutritional strategies to enhance education and productivity)* owes much to Commissioner Calloway and to Nevin Scrimshaw of MIT and the UNU; it draws on material from FAO 1985, UNACC/SCN 1987, Basta et al. 1979, Calloway 1982, Longhurst 1984, Popkin 1978, and Scrimshaw 1984. *Box 1.6 (The ratchet effect: a vicious cycle of illness and poverty)* is based largely on the work of Chambers 1989, Evans, T.G. 1989, and Zurbrigg 1984.

Chapter 2

From what is a substantial literature base about science and development and health research, the Commission drew upon the work of Abel-Smith and Creese 1989, Ballantyne 1984, Blumenfeld 1985, Campbell 1986, Clark 1977, Corning 1980, Lechat 1986, Mata and Rosero 1988, May et al. 1986, Nichols 1982, Pardey and Roseboom 1989, Rosenfield 1986,

Salam 1989, UNESCO 1986, Vuthipongse 1989, and Yeon 1989. The opinions and insights of researchers and policymakers from developing countries, especially those who participated in Commission workshops on essential national health research, constantly challenged the many drafts of this chapter and the opinions of the commissioners in its formulation. We are indebted to Richard Levins and Michael Reich for their careful critiques.

Material for *Box 2.1 (Smoking and health: a Chinese epidemic)* was contributed by J. Richard Bumgarner, China Department, the World Bank. *Box 2.2 (Social action in Bangladesh)* derives from Chowdhury et al. 1988a and b, and from the Bangladesh Rural Advancement Committee. *Box 2.3 (Smallpox: the global eradication of a disease)* was based primarily upon Fenner et al. 1988. *Box 2.4 (Malaria: intractability and the need for research)* is based upon Bruce-Chwatt 1985, UNDP/World Bank/WHO (TDR) 1989, and Kitron 1989. David J. Bradley at the London School of Hygiene and Tropical Medicine and Willy Piessens at the Harvard School of Public Health reviewed these boxes and other tropical disease materials. *Box 2.5 (AIDS orphans: social policy and action)* was based on field notes of Susan Hunter, a Rockefeller Foundation Fellow working at Makerere University, Kampala, Uganda, and David Hunter at the Harvard School of Public Health. *Box 2.6 (Recombinant DNA technology)* owes much to Piessens and the staff at Allelix, Inc., Ontario, and is also based on Darnell et al. 1986. *Box 2.7 (The promise of new vaccines)* was drafted by Julia Walsh (Harvard School of Public Health) and uses data from the Institute of Medicine 1984 and 1986. For *Box 2.8 (The cost-effectiveness of health research)*, we are indebted to Donald Shepard (Harvard School of Public Health and Harvard Institute of International Development); in addition, the box draws on the work of Abel-Smith and Creese 1989; Creese 1983, Ching 1988, Herrin and Rosenfield 1988 and the many valuable papers edited by them and produced for the Meeting on the Economics of Topical Diseases, Manila, Philippines, September 2-5, 1986; Shepard and Thompson 1979; Tugwell et al. 1984; and Westcott 1983. *Box 2.9 (Essential research for health in China)* was based on C.C. Chen 1989. *Box 2.10 (Essential health research in Mozambique)* derives from Cabral 1989 (contributed paper) and discussions at the Commission workshop on essential national research held in Zimbabwe. Materials for *Box 2.11 (Tuberculosis: a neglected disease)* include Styblo 1986; Murray, Styblo, and Rouillon 1989; Shimao 1989 (Commission paper); and WHO 1982. *Box 2.12 (Substance abuse: a global threat)* is based on work of WHO's Expert Committee on Drug Dependence 1989, Smart et al. 1985, Uchtenhagen 1986, and Aslam 1989 (staff paper).

Chapter 3

Chapter 3 is based predominantly on data collected and generated from the Commission survey of resources devoted to research on health problems of developing countries, described in the Commission paper by Murray et al. 1989. General data sources for the chapter include annual reports and budgetary information provided by development assistance agencies (public and private), foundations, industry, bilateral assistance institutions, and multinational organizations and their research programs, as well as health research institutions.

All are listed in the selected bibliography. The text also relies on Howard 1981, 1983; Howard 1989 (contributed paper); Lewis 1987; and Wheeler 1987.

Chapter 4

Health problems have been identified by numerous researchers, among whom the works of Briscoe et al. 1989; Lopez 1989; Walsh 1988; Mosley, Jamison, and Henderson 1990; Feachem, Murray, and Phillips 1990; Murray 1987; and Leslie and Buvinič 1989 (Commission paper) have been most relevant to our purposes. Discussions of health priorities and priority setting by Lopez and Ruzicka 1983; NEBT 1987; Walsh 1988; Walsh and Warren 1979 and 1986; U.S. Centers for Disease Control 1986; Rifkin 1985; Rifkin and Walt 1986; Fathalla 1988; and Feachem, Graham and Timaeus 1989 (Commission paper) informed the section on identifying and balancing priorities. Challenging and confirming our own assumptions about health research and action priorities were the many participants in essential national health research workshops, and contributors to the Commission country reports, listed in the selected bibliography.

Box 4.1 (Are post-transition diseases preventable?) was contributed by Commissioner Evans, based on Marmot and Theorell 1988. Box 4.2 (Contraception and reproductive health) is based on Mauldin and Segal 1988, Djerassi 1989, Fathalla 1988, and Germain and Ordway 1989. Box 4.3 (Deficiency of vitamin A: the quiet killer) is based on Berg and Brems 1986, and Sommer et al. 1983. Box 4.4 (Applied research on essential drugs) is based on the contributed paper of Ross-Degnan and Quick 1989. Material for Box 4.5 (Behavioral health in developing countries) was contributed by Kleinman and Eisenberg based on their own work and that of Hamburg et al. 1982; the box also derives from discussions at the Commission-sponsored workshop on behavioral problems affecting health in developing societies, November 28, 1988.

Chapter 5

The 10 Commission-sponsored country studies and the Commission's country workshops (held in Bangladesh, Brazil, Egypt, Mexico, and Zimbabwe as of this publication) provided material for this chapter. The country studies we commissioned are listed among country reports. The participants in and organizers of the Commission workshops were also important contributors and are included in the acknowledgments section of the book.

The chapter also owes credit to the following: Annerstedt and Jamison 1986, Blickenstaff and Moravcsik 1982, Brown et al. 1988, Cabral 1989 (contributed paper), Frame 1980, Gupta 1989, INCLEN 1988 (contributed paper), IDRC 1986, Martinez-Palomo and Sepulveda 1989, Poikolainen 1984, and the U.S. Department of Health and Human Services 1985.

Box 5.1 (Research capacity in case study countries) was generated from materials included in the country studies. Box 5.2 (Mexico: a special program for national research) is based on Malo and Gonzalez 1988, Malo 1988, Garza and Malo 1988. Material for Box 5.3 (Linking researchers and policymakers in the Philippines) was contributed by Mario Feranil of PIDS. Box 5.4 (Shaping medical education to country-specific health needs) derives from material contributed by Vic Neufeld of the Network of Community-Oriented Educational Institutions for Health Sciences and by Commissioner Lucas. Box 5.5 (The Third World Academy of Sciences) is based on the academy's 1989 yearbook.

Chapter 6

The data in this chapter are primarily from OECD 1981 and 1985, IMF 1988, IDRC 1986, and BOSTID/IOM 1987. The chapter discussion of industrialized-country research on health problems of developing countries is based on Advisory Council for Scientific Research in Development Problems 1984, Henderson 1987 (Commission paper), Fogarty International Center 1987, Mosley and Mauck 1988, Rifkin 1989 (staff paper), Smuckler et al. 1988, and UNFPA 1988. Discussion of international research centers is based on Corning 1980; ICD-DR,B 1986; and IDRC 1987. The discussion of the Consultative Group on International Agricultural Research (CGIAR) is based on a variety of CGIAR publications listed as CGIAR 1985, 1986, and 1987, Baum 1986, and Bell 1989 (staff paper).

References throughout the chapter to the European tropical research institutes, summarized in Box 6.1 (The future role of European tropical institutes) owe much to ideas expressed by participants at the Commission-sponsored workshop addressing these issues held in Amsterdam, November 31–December 1, 1989. Box 6.2 (Japan's international cooperation in health) derives from Okita 1989 (Commission paper), Shimao 1989 (Commission paper), and Wagatsuma 1989 (contributed paper), supplemented by comments from Shigekoto Kaihara and Eiji Marui. Box 6.3 (Viral diseases: early recognition of shared health threats) was contributed by Commissioner Evans. Box 6.4 (Private initiatives for tropical disease research) is based on recent annual reports from the Rockefeller, MacArthur, and Clark foundations. Lastly, Box 6.5 (A Latin American initiative for regional vaccine research and development) is based on materials provided by Commissioner Martinez-Palomo.

Chapter 7

The observations on the role of multilateral and bilateral agencies derive from the WHO Office of Research Promotion and Development 1988; the WHO Division of Strengthening of Health Services, Programme on Health Systems Research and Development 1988; the WHO Advisory Committee on Health Research 1986; the International Development Research Centre 1986, the UNDP/World Bank/WHO Special Programme for Research and Training in Tropical Diseases (TDR) 1989; the UNDP/UNFPA/World Bank/WHO Special Programme of Research, Development and Research Training in Human Reproduction (HRP) 1988; the WHO Programme for Control of Diarrhoeal Diseases 1988; and Winrock International 1988. The discussion of international research promotion activities by foundations is based on a substantial body of information provided to the Commission from philanthropic foundations, including publications or personal communication from the Aga Khan Foundation, the Carnegie Corporation, the Edna McConnell Clark Foundation, the Ford Foundation, the John D. and Catherine T. MacArthur Foundation, the Pew Charitable Trusts, the Rockefeller Foundation, the Sasakawa Memorial Health Foundation, and the Wellcome Trust, all listed fully by organization in the selected bibliography. Lastly, the work of Lewis 1987 was used in writing this chapter.

Box 7.1 (Two WHO-associated research programs: HRP and TDR) is based on publications of those programs and the views of Commissioner Bergstrom. *Box 7.2 (Research on onchocerciasis)* was contributed by Bernhard Liese of the World Bank and OCP. *Box 7.3 (Industry collaboration in research on developing-country health problems)* is based on Blair 1988 and the UNDP/World Bank/WHO (TDR) 1989. *Box 7.4 (Debate over intellectual property rights)* is based on the work of the Overseas Development Council 1989. Lastly, materials contributed from Robbins and Freeman, and their 1988 publication, form the basis for *Box 7.5 (Front-end funding for vaccine development)*.

Chapter 8

The Chapter 8 discussion of research capacity building draws upon the work of many researchers, including Brown et al. 1988; Dow 1988; Evans 1981; Faundes 1988 (contributed paper); Freij and Oliw 1986 (contributed paper); Ghai 1974; Gupta 1989 (contributed paper); Harkavy and Diescho 1989 (Commission paper); Hughes and Hunter 1970; ICDDR,B 1989; INCLEN 1988; IDRC 1987; Scrimshaw 1989; annual reports of TDR and HRP; and Weisblat and Kearl 1989.

Box 8.1 (Building capacity for demographic research in China) is based on Greenhalgh 1988. *Box 8.2 (Newer foundation programs to support capacity building)* is based on personal communication with Dr. Ronald Wilson of the Aga Khan Foundation and publications of the Sasakawa Memorial Health Foundation (1988) and the Pew Charitable Trusts (1987). *Box 8.3 (Research capacity building by IDRC and SAREC)* is based on IDRC 1987 and SAREC 1987. *Box 8.4 (Building epidemiological and field research capacities: the TDR experience)* was contributed by Richard Morrow of TDR. *Box 8.5 (A regional individual awards program in the Middle East)* is based on Harkavy and Diescho 1989 (Commission paper). Scrimshaw 1989 forms the basis of *Box 8.6 (Building nutritional research capacity: INCAP and UNU)*. *Box 8.7 (Regional networking: the SEAMEO-TROPMED model)* is based on materials contributed by Dr. Chamlong Harinasuta in 1988 and SEAMEO-TROPMED 1989. Lastly, *Box 8.8 (Human and institutional development in Africa)* was contributed in part by Dr. Aklilu Lemma of the ICDC, and is in part based on discussions with David DeFerranti and other World Bank officials.

Working Papers

COUNTRY REPORTS

Bangladesh
Abed, F.H. 1988. "Health Research Capacities in Bangladesh—Some Observations." Bangladesh Rural Advancement Committee, Dhaka.

Rahman, O. 1990. "Health Research in Bangladesh." Discussion paper. Bangladesh Institute for Development Studies, Dhaka.

Brazil
Carvalho da Silva, A. 1989 (July). "Health research in Brazil." A report for the Commission on Health Research for Development. São Paulo.

Marques, M.B., C. Possas, P. Buss, H. Cordeiro. 1989 (October). "Health Research in Brazil." Rio de Janeiro.

Egypt
Ezzat, E. 1989 (August). "Health-Related Research in Egypt." Suez Canal University Medical School, Ismailia.

———. 1988. "Enhancing Capacity for Health Research in Developing Countries—Egyptian Perspective." Suez Canal University Medical School, Ismailia.

Waheeb, Y. 1989 (December). "Country Case Study: Health Research in Egypt." Faculty of Medicine, Suez Canal University, Ismailia.

Ethiopia
Habte, D. 1988. "The State of Health Research in Ethiopa." Addis Ababa University, Addis Ababa.

Kebede, D. 1989. "Country-specific and Transnational Health Research in Ethiopia." Department of Community Health, Addis Ababa University, Addis Ababa.

India
Murthy, N. and N.S. Deodhar. 1989 (November). "Financing of Health Research in India." Research Report, Public Systems Group, Indian Institute of Management, Ahmedabad.

Ramalingaswami, V. 1988 (May). "Health Research Capability Building." UNICEF, New York.

Uplekar, M. 1990 (in preparation). "Health Research in India." Foundation for Research in Community Health, Bombay.

Mali
Koita, A. 1989 (July). "Financement de la Recherche Sanitaire au Mali." Institut de Santé Publique, Bamako.

Pearce, M. 1989 (December). "Health Research in Mali." London School of Hygiene and Tropical Medicine, London.

Mexico
Bobadilla, J., J. Frenk, and J. Sepulveda. 1988. "Health Research in Mexico: Strengths, Weaknesses and Gaps." Background paper prepared for the Commission on Health Research for Development. Mexico City.

Cruz, C., E. del Carmen Sanchez, and B. Hernandez. 1989 (July). "Resources for Health Research in Mexico." Background paper prepared for the Commission on Health Research for Development. National Institute of Public Health, Cuernavaca.

Hernandez, M. and J. Sepulveda. "Health Research in Mexico." Background paper for the regional Central-American workshop on health information and research. Puebla, Mexico. January 18-19, 1990.

Nigeria
Lucas, A.O. 1988. "Medical Research in Nigeria." Carnegie Corporation, New York.

Ministry of Health, Nigeria. 1987 (December). "The National Health Policy and Strategy to Achieve Health for All Nigerians."

Philippines
Baltazar, J. and M.M.L. Quesada. 1988. "Enhancing Capacity for Health Research: The Philippine Experience." College of Public Health, University of the Philippines, Manila.

Zara, P. 1989 (July). "Health Research Resources in the Philippines." Philippine Council for Health Research and Development, Manila.

Thailand
Kaewsonthi, S. 1989 (June). "Resources for Health Research in Thailand." Chulalongkorn University, Bangkok.

Sornmani, S. 1988 (May). "Research on the Application of Health Concepts and Tools in Developing Countries with Special Emphasis on Southeast Asia." Faculty of Tropical Medicine, Mahidol University, Bangkok.

Zimbabwe
Kamba, W.J. 1988 (May). "Health Research in Zimbabwe: Problems and Strategies for Development." University of Zimbabwe, Harare.

Loewenson, R., M. Mhloyi, and S. Tswana. 1989 (August). "Essential National Research for Health and Development: A Situation Analysis in Zimbabwe." University of Zimbabwe, Harare.

University of Zimbabwe. 1988 (January). "Report of Health and Medical Research Carried Out in Zimbabwe." University of Zimbabwe, Harare.

COMMISSION PAPERS

Abel-Smith, B. 1989. "Health Economics in Developing Countries. " *Journal of Tropical Medicine and Hygiene* 92:229-41.

Bhatia, S., F. Saadah, and W.H. Mosley. 1989 (January). "Analytical Review of the Development of Family Planning Program Strategies, Operations, and Research as a Model for Primary Health Care Programs." The Johns Hopkins University School of Hygiene and Public Health, Baltimore.

Cairncross, S. 1989. "Water Supply and Sanitation." *Journal of Tropical Medicine and Hygiene* 92:301-14.

Chen, L.C. 1988. "Ten Years after Alma-Ata: Balancing Different Primary Health Care Strategies." State of the Art Lecture. 12th International Congress for Tropical Medicine and Malaria, Amsterdam. *Tropical and Geographical Medicine* 40, 3:S-22-9.

Chen, L.C. and R.A. Cash. 1988. "A Decade after Alma-Ata: Can Primary Health Care Lead to Health for All?" *The New England Journal of Medicine* 319:946-47.

Evans, J.R. 1989 (April). "Health Research: Essential or Marginal to Health for All?" Michael Wood Memorial Lecture, African Medical and Research Foundation, Nairobi.

Evans, J.R. 1988. "Health Research for Development." Keynote Address, 12th International Congress for Tropical Medicine and Malaria, Amsterdam. *Tropical and Geographical Medicine,* 40, 3:S2-5.

Feachem, R.G., W.J. Graham, and I. Timaeus. 1989. "Identifying Health Problems and Health Research Priorities in Developing Countries." London School of Hygiene and Tropical Medicine, London. *Journal of Tropical Medicine and Hygiene* 92, 3:133-91.

Gust, I. 1989. "Hepatitus B." Royal Fairfield Hospital, Melbourne.

Habte, D. 1989. "The Crisis of Child Health in Developing Countries." Addis Ababa University, Addis Ababa.

Harkavy, O., and L. Diescho. 1989. "Lessons from Donor Experience in Capacity Strengthening for Health Research in the Developing World." Commission on Health Research for Development, Cambridge, Mass.

Henderson, D.A. 1987 (July). "Application and Problem Solving in Health Research for the Developing Countries." The Johns Hopkins University School of Hygiene and Public Health, Baltimore, Md.

Kleinman, A., and J. Sugar. 1988 (November). "Report on the Workshop on Behaviorial Conditions in International Health." Commission on Health Research for Development, Cambridge, Mass.

Murray, C.J.L., D.E. Bell, E. De Jonghe, C. Michaud, and S. Zaidi. 1989. "A Study of Financial Resources Devoted to Research on Health Problems of Developing Countries." Commission on Health Research for Development, Cambridge, Mass.

Leslie, J., and M. Buvinic. 1989 (July). "Strengthening Women: Health Research Priorities for Women in Developing Countries." International Center for Research on Women, Washington D.C.

Okita, S. 1989 (June). "Japan and Third World Development." III World Scientific Banking Meeting, Dubrovnik.

————. 1989. "Japan's Growing Role for Development Financing." In *International Cooperation for Health: Problems, Prospects, and Priorities,* edited by M.R. Reich and E. Marui. Dover, Mass.: Auburn House.

Philips, M. 1989. "Health Economics Research—Report of a Meeting Held on Behalf of the Commission on Health Research for Development." London School of Hygiene and Tropical Medicine, London. *Health Policy and Planning* 2.

Shimao, T. 1989. "Institutional Capacity for Disease-Research and Control: The Case of Tuberculosis." In *International Cooperation for Health: Problems, Prospects, and Priorities,* edited by M.R. Reich and E. Marui. Dover, Mass.: Auburn House.

STAFF PAPERS

Aslam, A. 1989. "Heroinization of Pakistan." Commission on Health Research for Development, Cambridge, Mass.

Bell, D.E. 1989 (March). "Possible Lessons from International Research Institutions in Agriculture for Health Research." Commission on Health Research for Development, Cambridge, Mass.

Bell, D.E., and C. Nelson. 1987 (July). "How Well Do Present Research and Development Activities Address Critical Health Problems of Developing Countries?" Commission on Health Research for Development, Cambridge, Mass.

Castillo, G.T. 1988 (April). "Health Policy Research: Some General Issues." Paper prepared for the First Meeting of the International Health Policy Program, Nairobi.

Evans, J.R. 1988. "Improving Health Research for Developing Countries." Commission on Health Research for Development, Cambridge, Mass.

Hoskins, E. 1988 (September). "Refugee Health." London School of Hygiene and Tropical Medicine, London.

Mukharji, D. 1987 (July). "Research Priorities for Effective Community-based Action in Health." Christian Medical Association of India, Nagpur.

Murray, C.J.L. 1988 (January). "A Conceptual Framework for Establishing Health Priorities." Commission on Health Research for Development, Cambridge, Mass.

Myers, J., R. Durvasula, and D. Christiani. 1988 (June). "Report and Review of Research Needs in the Field of Occupational Health with Special Reference to Developing Countries." Commission on Health Research for Development, Cambridge, Mass.

Nelson, C. 1987 (December). "Support for Capacity-Building in the Third World." Commission on Health Research for Development, Cambridge, Mass.

Peterson, K. 1988 (December). "Report on the Workshop on Micronutrient Deficiencies." Commission on Health Research for Development, Cambridge, Mass.

Reich, M.R., and C. Palmer. 1988 (November). "Smoking and Health in the Developing Countries." Commission on Health Research for Development, Cambridge, Mass.

Rifkin, S. 1989 (April). "Review of Selected European Research Institutions and Funding Bodies for Health Research in Developing Countries." Liverpool School of Tropical Medicine, Liverpool.

Shrinivasa-Murthy, R. 1989 (January). "Mental Health." National Institute of Mental Health and Neuro Sciences, Bangalore.

Tanner, M. 1988 (May). "District-level Data Collection and Use." Swiss Tropical Institute, Basel.

Walsh, J.A., and V. Ramalingaswami. 1987 (July). "Biomedical Research: Status and Opportunities." Commission on Health Research for Development, Cambridge, Mass.

CONTRIBUTED PAPERS

Addis Ababa University Faculty of Medicine and Karolinska Institute. 1987 (November). "Development of Biomedical Research Training in Ethiopia." Addis Ababa.

Argandona-Yanez, M. 1988 (November). "Alcoholism and Alcohol-Related Problems in Developing Societies." Prepared for the Workshop on Behavioral Problems Affecting Health in Developing Societies. Commission on Health Research for Development, Cambridge, Mass.

Cabral, A.J.R. 1989 (August). "Essential National Health Research—A Perspective from the South." Paper presented at the Commission workshop on essential national health information and research in Harare, Ministry of Health, Maputo.

Carrin, G. 1988 (April). "Concise Overview of Work in the EEC on Health Policy in Developing Countries." School of Tropical Medicine, Antwerp.

Earls, F. 1988 (November). "Approaches to the Expansion of Mental Health Services for Children in Developing Countries." Harvard School of Public Health, Boston.

Eisenberg, L. 1988 (November). "Failures Resulting from Success." Paper prepared for the Workshop on Behavioral Problems Affecting Health in Developing Societies. Commission on Health Research for Development, Cambridge, Mass.

Faundes, A. 1988. "Enhancing Capacity for Health Research in Developing Countries." University of Campinas, Campinas.

Freij, L., and E. Oliw, eds. 1986 (September). "Development Cooperation in the Field of Health Research Training—A Report from a Study Tour to Pakistan, Bangladesh, Somalia, Ethiopia and Zimbabwe Jointly Organised by SAREC and the Karolinska Institute." Report for a SAREC workshop, Saltsjobaden.

Frenk, J., J.L. Bobadilla, J. Sepulveda, and M.L. Cervantes. 1989. "Health Transition in Middle Income Countries: New Challenges for Health Care." *Health Policy and Planning* 4, 1:29-39.

Gupta, P. 1989. "International Cooperation in Dealing with Health Problems Caused by Tobacco." In *International Cooperation for Health: Problems, Prospects, and Priorities*, edited by M.R. Reich and E. Marui. Dover, Mass. Auburn House.

Hollifield, M. 1988 (November). "Psychiatry in Developing Countries, Evidence of the Burden and Intervention Efficacy in Primary Care." Draft presented at the Workshop on the Behavioral Problems Affecting Health in Developing Societies. Commission on Health Research for Development, Cambridge, Mass.

Howard, L. 1989. "The Evolution of Bilateral and Multilateral Cooperation for Health in Developing Countries." In *International Cooperation for Health: Problems, Prospects, and Priorities*, edited by M.R. Reich and E. Marui. Dover, Mass.: Auburn House.

International Clinical Epidemiology Network (INCLEN). 1988 (November). "Recommendations to the Commission." Commission on Health Research for Development, Cambridge, Mass.

Ishikawa, N. 1989 (June). "BRAC's Tuberculosis Program." The Research Institute of Tuberculosis, Kiyose. Paper presented to the Commission on Health Research for Development, Satellite Session, Kiyose.

Johnston, L.D. 1988 (November). "Illicit Drug Use: Problems and Needs at the World Level." Paper prepared for Workshop on Behaviorial Conditions in International Health. University of Michigan, Ann Arbor.

Kleinman, A. 1988 (November). "Psychosocial and Psychiatric Conditions in Primary Health Care in Developing Societies." Paper prepared for the Workshop on Behaviorial Conditions in International Health. Commission on Health Research for Development, Cambridge, Mass.

Loewenson, R. 1988 (January). "Research in the Faculty of Medicine: Problems and Strategies for Development." Paper presented to the Commission on Health Research for Development, Harare.

Mati, J.K.G. 1988 (January). "Health Research Needs for Africa." Paper presented to the Commission on Health Research for Development, Harare.

Max, E. 1989. "Leprosy Control in India: International Cooperation." In *International Cooperation for Health: Problems, Prospects, and Priorities*, edited by M.R. Reich and E. Marui. Dover, Mass.: Auburn House.

Metcalfe, S. 1988 (January). "Health Research Activities from the Perspective of NGOs." Paper presented to the Commission on Health Research for Development, Harare.

Mhloyi, M.M. 1988 (January). "Health Research for Development: A Social Science Perspective." Paper presented to the Commission on Health Research for Development, Harare.

Muhondwa, E.P.Y. 1989. "The Role and Impact of Foreign Aid in Tanzania's Health Development." In *International Cooperation for Health: Problems, Prospects, and Priorities*, edited by M.R. Reich and E. Marui. Dover, Mass.: Auburn House.

Murthy, R.S. 1988. "Mental Health in Developing Countries—Needs, Priorities, and Approaches." Commission on Health Research for Development, Cambridge, Mass.

Mutambirwa, J. 1988 (January). "User Perspectives in Health Activities and Application of Health Research in Developing Countries." Paper presented to the Commission on Health Research for Development, Harare.

Nhonoli, A.M. 1988. "Priorities for Health Research in the Region." Paper presented to the Commission on Health Research for Development, Commonwealth Regional Health Secretariat, Arusha.

Ramalingaswami, P. 1989 (July). "Social Sciences and Health in India." Jawaharlal Nehru University, New Delhi.

Ramesh, J. 1988 (December). "Charkha, Chip and Community: The Technology Missions." Planning Commission, Government of India.

Ross-Degnan, D., and J. Quick. 1989. "Research Priorities for Promoting Effective Drug Utilization." Commission on Health Research for Development, Cambridge, Mass.

Samarasinghe, S.W.R. 1989. "Japanese and U.S. Health Assistance to Sri Lanka." In *International Cooperation for Health: Problems, Prospects, and Priorities*, edited by M.R. Reich and E. Marui. Dover, Mass.: Auburn House.

Sartorius, N. 1988 (November). "Cross-cultural and International Collaboration in Mental Health Research and Action: Experience from the Mental Health Programme of the World Health Organization." Paper presented at the Workshop on Behavioral Problems Affecting Health in Developing Societies, World Health Organization, Geneva.

Sikipa, G.G. 1988 (January). "Health Research for Development." Paper presented to the Commission on Health Research for Development, Harare.

Wagatsuma, T. 1989. "Department of International Cooperation and Its Future Role in Japan's Development Assistance." In *International Cooperation for Health: Problems, Prospects, and Priorities*, edited by M.R. Reich and E. Marui. Dover, Mass.: Auburn House.

SELECTED BIBLIOGRAPHY

Abel-Smith, B. 1978. *Poverty, Development and Health Policy.* Geneva: World Health Organization (WHO).

Abel-Smith, B., and A. Creese, eds. 1989. *Recurrent Costs in the Health Sector—Problems and Policy Options in Three Countries.* Geneva: WHO.

Action Programme on Essential Drugs. 1988. *The World Drug Situation.* Geneva: WHO.

Administration Générale de la Coopération au Développement. 1988. *La Belgique et la Coopération au Développement.* Brussels: AGCD.

Advisory Committee on Health Research. 1986. *Health Research Strategy.* Geneva: WHO.

Advisory Committee on Health Research. 1986.[a] "Enhancement of Transfer of Technology to Developing Countries with Special Reference to Health." Report of a Subcommittee of the ACHR. Geneva: WHO.

Advisory Council for Scientific Research in Development Problems (RAWOO). 1984. *Health and Illness in Developing Countries: Research Needs and Priorities.* Netherlands: RAWOO.

Aga Khan Foundation. 1989. "Institutional Capacity to Address Health Problems." In *International Cooperation for Health: Problems, Prospects, and Priorities,* edited by M.R. Reich and E. Marui. Dover, Mass: Auburn House.

Albanez, T., E. Bustelo, G.A. Cornia, and E. Jespersen. 1989. *Economic Decline and Child Survival: The Plight of Latin America in the Eighties.* Innocenti Occasional Papers, No. 1 (March). Florence, Italy: UNICEF International Child Development Centre.

Alleyne, G.A.O. 1989. "Health and Development: Caribbean Perspectives." Seventh lecture in the Dr. Eric Williams Memorial Lecture Series. Port of Spain, Trinidad and Tobago: Central Bank of Trinidad and Tobago.

Annerstedt, J., and A. Jamison. 1986. *Science and Technology for Development: Scandinavian Efforts to Foster Development Research and Transfer Resources for Research and Experimental Development to Developing Countries.* Paris: United Nations Educational, Scientific and Cultural Organization (UNESCO).

Australian International Development Assistance Bureau. 1986. *A Profile of the Health Sector in Australian Development Assistance.* Sectoral Studies Section, Australian International Development Assistance Bureau.

Ballantyne, A.O. 1984. "Agriculture Research and the Developing Country." *World Crops* (November-December): 196-98.

Bangladesh Rural Advancement Committee. 1989. "Controlling a Forgotten Disease: The Case of Tuberculosis in a Primary Health Care Setting in Rural Bangladesh." Dhaka: BRAC.

Basta, S., M. Soekirman, D. Karyadi, and N. Scrimshaw. 1979. "Iron Deficiency Anemia and the Productivity of Adult Males in Indonesia." *American Journal of Clinical Nutrition* 32:916-25.

Baum, W.C. 1986. *Partners Against Hunger: The Consultative Group on International Agricultural Research.* Washington, D.C.: World Bank.

Behrman, J. 1988. "The Impact of Economic Adjustment Programs." In *Health, Nutrition, and Economic Crises,* edited by D. Bell and M. Reich. Dover, Mass.: Auburn House.

Bell, D.E., and Reich M.R., eds. 1988. *Health, Nutrition and Economic Crises.* Dover, Mass.: Auburn House.

Berg, A., and S. Brems. 1986 (December). *Micronutrient Deficiencies: Present Knowledge on Effects and Control.* Population, Health, and Nutrition Department. Washington, D.C.: World Bank.

Better Health Through Family Planning. 1987. Recommendations of the International Conference on Better Health for Women and Children Through Family Planning. Nairobi, Kenya.

Bhopal Working Group. 1987. "The Public Health Implications of the Bhopal Disaster." *American Journal of Public Health* 77, 2:230-36.

Birdsall, N. 1989. "Thoughts on Good Health and Good Government." *Daedalus* 118 (Winter) 1:89-123.

Blair, K. 1988 (November) *Industry Report.* Donaldson, Lufkin, and Jenrette, Inc: Datext.

Blickenstaff, J., and M.J. Moravcsik. 1982. "Scientific Output in the Third World." *Scientometrics* 4, 2:135-69.

Blumenfeld, S. 1985. "Operations Research Methods: A General

Approach in Primary Health Care." Chevy Chase, Md.: Primary Health Care Operations Research, Center for Human Services.

Board on Science and Technology for International Development (BOSTID) and Institute of Medicine (IOM). 1987. *The U.S. Capacity to Address Tropical Infectious Disease Problems.* Washington, D.C.: National Academy Press.

Bradley, D.J. 1977. "The Health Implications of Irrigation Schemes and Man-Made Lakes in Tropical Environments." In *Water, Wastes and Health in Hot Climates,* edited by R. Feachem, M. McGarry, and D. Mara. London: John A. Wiley.

Brandt Commission. 1985. *Common Crisis North-South: Cooperation for World Recovery.* Cambridge, Mass.: MIT Press.

Briscoe, J., A.C. Campos, and N. Birdsall. 1989. *Adult Health in Brazil: Adjusting to New Challenges.* Washington, D.C.: World Bank.

Brokensha, D., K. MacQueen, and L. Stress. 1988. *Anthropological Perspectives on AIDS in Africa: Priorities for Intervention and Research.* Binghamton, N.Y.: Institute for Development Anthropology.

Brown, G., A.K. Jain, and B. Gyepi-Garbrah. 1988. "Review of Institutional Capacities and Human Resources in Population and Reproductive Health in Sub-Saharan Africa." Paper prepared for the meeting on "Institutional Development in Population and Reproductive Health in Sub-Saharan Africa." Saly Portadal, Senegal, November 1988. New York: Population Council.

Brown, L. 1989. *State of the World 1989. A Worldwatch Institute Report on Progress Toward a Sustainable Society.* New York/London: W.W. Norton.

Bruce-Chwatt, L.J. 1985. *Essential Malariology.* 2nd ed. London: William Heinemann Medical Books.

Bulatao, R., A. Lopez, P. Stephens. 1989 (draft). "Estimates and Projections of Mortality by Cause: A Global Overview, 1970-2015." In *Evolving Health Sector Priorities in Developing Countries,* edited by D. Jamison and W. Henry Mosley. Population, Health and Nutrition Division, The World Bank. Washington, D.C.: World Bank.

Caldwell, J.C., and P. Caldwell. 1989. "Changing Health Conditions." In *International Cooperation for Health: Problems, Prospects, and Priorities,* edited by M.R. Reich and E. Marui. Dover, Mass: Auburn House.

Calloway, D.H. 1982. "Functional Consequences of Malnutri-

tion." *Reviews of Infectious Diseases* 4:736-45.

Campbell, F. 1986. "The Role of Research in Third World Development." *With Our Own Hands: Research for Third World Development: Canada's Contribution Through the International Development Research Centre 1970-1985.* Ottawa: International Development Research Centre (IDRC).

Canadian International Development Agency. 1987. *Annual Report 1986-1987.* Quebec: IDRC.

Carnegie Corporation of New York. 1986. *Annual Report 1986.* New York: Carnegie Corporation.

Chambers, R., ed. 1989. "Vulnerability: How the Poor Cope." *IDS Bulletin 20* (April) 2.

Chen, C.C., in collaboration with Frederica M. Bunge. 1989. *Medicine in Rural China: A Personal Account.* Berkeley: University of California Press.

Chen, L.C. 1986. "Primary Health Care in Developing Countries: Overcoming Operational, Technical, and Social Barriers." *The Lancet* (Nov.) 29:1260-65.

Children's Defense Fund. 1989. *A Vision for America's Future—An Agenda for the 1990s: A Children's Defense Budget.* Washington, D.C.: Children's Defense Fund.

Ching, P. 1988. "Some Key Issues on the Economics of Tropical Diseases." *Economics, Health and Tropical Diseases.* Manila: University of the Philippines School of Economics.

Chowdhury, A.M.R., F. Karim, and J. Ahmed. 1988. "Teaching ORT to Women: Individually or in Groups?" *Journal of Tropical Medicine and Hygiene* 91:283-87.

Chowdhury, A.M.R., J.P. Vaughan, and F.H. Abed. 1988. "Use and Safety of Home-Made Oral Rehydration Solutions: an Epidemiological Evaluation from Bangladesh." *International Journal of Epidemiology* 17, 3:655-65.

Edna McConnell Clark Foundation. 1986. *1986 Annual Report—October 1, 1985 - September 30, 1986.* New York: EMCF.

Clark, G. 1977. *World Prehistory in New Perspective.* London: Cambridge University Press.

Consultative Group on International Agricultural Research. 1987. *Annual Report 1986-87.* Washington, D.C.: CGIAR Secretariat.

———. 1986. *Report of the External Program Review of the International Service for National Agricultural Research* (ISNAR).

Rome: Technical Advisory Committee Secretariat, Food and Agricultural Organization (FAO).

———. 1985. *International Agricultural Research Centers: A Study of Achievements and Potential.* Washington, D.C.: World Bank.

Cornia, G.A., R. Jolly, and F. Stewart, eds. 1987. *Adjustment with a Human Face:* Vol. 1.—*Protecting the Vulnerable and Promoting Growth*; Vol. 2—*Country Case Studies.* New York: Oxford University Press.

Corning, M. 1980. *A Review of the United States Role in International Biomedical Research and Communications.* Bethesda, Md.: U.S. Department of Health and Human Services, National Institutes of Health.

Creese, A. 1983. "The Economic Evaluation of Immunization Programmes." In *The Economics of Health in Developing Countries,* edited by K. Lee and A. Mills. Oxford: Oxford University Press.

Danish International Development Agency (DANIDA). 1987. *Denmark's Development Assistance.* DANIDA, Ministry of Foreign Affairs.

Darnell, J.E., H.F. Lodish, and D. Baltimore. 1986. *Molecular Cell Biology.* New York: Scientific American Books.

Deutsche Gesellschaft für Technische Zusammenarbeit (GTZ). 1986.[a] *Annual Report 1985.* Eschborn: GTZ.

———.[b] *Key Services: Development of Basic Medical Services, Central Medical Services, Nutrition.* Eschborn: GTZ.

Direzione Generale per la Cooperazione allo Sviluppo. 1989[a]. *La Cooperazione Sanitaria Italiana: Rapporto Annuale 1988.* Rome: Ministero Degli Affari Esteri.

———. 1989[b]. *La Cooperazione Sanitaria Italiana: Principi Guida.* Rome: Ministero Degli Affari Esteri.

Djerassi, C. 1989. "The Bitter Pill." *Science* 245:245-361.

Dow, M. 1988 (Summer). "Scientific Institution-Building in Africa." *BOSTID Developments* 8, 1.

Eisenberg, L. 1987. "Preventing Mental, Neurological and Psychosocial Disorders." *World Health Forum* 8:1-9.

Evans, J., K.I. Hall, and J. Warford. 1981. "Shattuck Lecture on Health Care in the Developing World: Problems of Scarcity and Choice." *New England Journal of Medicine,* 305, 19:1117-27.

Evans, J. 1988. "Health Research for Development." *Tropical and Geographical Medicine* 40, 3:S2-S5 (Supplement).

———. 1981. *Measurement and Management in Health Services: Training Needs and Opportunities.* New York: Rockefeller Foundation.

Evans, T.G. 1989. "The Impact of Permanent Disability on Rural Households: River Blindness in Guinea." *IDS Bulletin* 20 (April) 2:41-48.

Fathalla, M.F. 1988. "Research Needs in Human Reproduction." In *Research in Human Reproduction: Biennial Report 1986-87,* edited by E. Diczfalusy, P.D. Griffin, and J. Khanna. Geneva: WHO.

Feachem, R.G., C. Murray, and M.A. Phillips. 1990 (forthcoming). T*he Health of Adults in the Developing World.* Washington, D.C.: World Bank.

Fenner, F., D.A. Henderson, I. Arita, Z. Jezek, and I.D. Kadnyi. 1988. *Smallpox and Its Eradication.* Geneva: WHO.

Fogarty International Center for Advanced Study in the Health Sciences. 1987. *National Institutes of Health Annual Report of International Activities—Fiscal Year 1987.* Washington, D.C.: U.S. Department of Health and Human Services, National Institutes of Health.

Food and Agriculture Organization of the United Nations (FAO). 1985. *Fifth World Food Survey.* Rome: FAO.

———. 1984. *Integrating Nutrition into Agricultural and Rural Development Projects: Six Case Studies.* Nutrition in Agriculture Series, No. 2. Rome: FAO.

The Ford Foundation. 1987. *Annual Report 1986.* New York: Ford Foundation.

Frame, J.D. 1980. "Measuring Scientific Activity in Lesser Developed Countries." *Scientometrics* 2, 2:133-45.

Frame, J.D., and F. Narin. 1987. "The Growth of Chinese Scientific Research." *Scientometrics* 12, 1-2:134-44.

Garza, G., and S. Malo. 1988. "La formación académica de los investigadores." *Ciencia y Desarrollo* 14, 82:93-102.

Germain, A., and J. Ordway. 1989. *Population Control and Women's Health: Balancing the Scales.* New York: International Women's Health Coalition in Cooperation with the Overseas Development Council.

Ghai, D. 1974. "Social Science Research on Development and

Research Institutes in Africa." Paper presented at "Social Science Research on Development" seminar. Bellagio, Italy, February 1974. Kenya: Institute for Development Studies, University of Nairobi.

Ghana Health Assessment Project Team. 1981. "A Quantitative Method of Assessing the Health Impact of Different Diseases in Less Developed Countries." *International Journal of Epidemiology* 10, 1:73-80.

Gopalan, C. 1989. "Science and Nutrition in the Future." Plenary Lecture, 14th International Congress of Nutrition. Seoul, South Korea, August 22, 1989.

Greenhalgh, S. 1988. "Population Research in China: An Introduction and Guide to Institutes." Working Paper No. 137, Center for Policy Studies. New York: Population Council.

Halstead, S.B. 1988. "International Clinical Epidemiology Network." Information Sheet, INCLEN. New York: Rockefeller Foundation.

Halstead, S.B., J.A. Walsh, and K.S. Warren, eds. 1985. *Good Health at Low Cost*. New York: Rockefeller Foundation.

Hamburg, et al., eds. 1982. *Health and Behavior: Frontiers of Research in the Biobehavioral Sciences*. Division of Mental Health and Behavioral Medicine, Institute of Medicine. Washington, D.C.: National Academy of Sciences.

Herrin, A.N., and P.L. Rosenfield, eds. 1988.[a] *Economics, Health and Tropical Diseases*. Papers, Summary and Conclusions of the Meeting on the Economics of Tropical Diseases. Manila, Philippines, September 2-5, 1986. Manila: University of the Philippines School of Economics.

———.1988.[b] "The Economics of Tropical Diseases: Issues and Research Directions." *Economics, Health and Tropical Diseases*. Manila: University of the Philippines School of Economics.

Herz, B., and A.R. Measham. 1987. *The Safe Motherhood Initiative: Proposals for Action*. Washington, D.C.: World Bank.

William and Flora Hewlett Foundation. 1987. *1987 Annual Report*. Menlo Park, Calif.: William and Flora Hewlett Foundation.

Howard, L. 1983. "International Sources of Financial Cooperation for Health in Developing Countries." *Bulletin of the Pan American Health Organization* 17, 2.

———. 1981. *A New Look at Development Cooperation for Health: A Study of Official Donor Policies, Programmes, and*

Perspectives in Support of Health for All by the Year 2000. Geneva: WHO.

Huddle, N., and M. Reich with N. Stiskin. 1987. *Island of Dreams: Environmental Crisis in Japan*. Rochester, Vt.: Schenkman Books.

Hughes, C.C., and J.M. Hunter. 1970. "Disease and 'Development' in Africa." *Social Science and Medicine* 3:443-93.

Independent Commission on International Humanitarian Issues. 1988. *Winning the Human Race?* London/New Jersey: Zed Books.

Ingram, G.K. 1989. "Economic Development: Its Record and Determinants." Prepared for the World Management Congress. New York, September 1989. Washington, D.C.: World Bank.

Institut de Médecine Tropicale Prince Leopold. 1986. *Rapport annuel 1985-1986*. Antwerp, Belgium: ITG IMT.

Institut Français de Recherche Scientifique pour le Développement en Coopération (ORSTOM). 1987. *Rapport de la Septième Session du Conseil de Département*. Paris: ORSTOM.

Institute of Medicine. 1984 and 1986. *New Vaccine Development: Establishing Priorities*; Vol. 1: *Diseases of Importance in the United States*; and Vol. 2: *Diseases of Importance in Developing Countries*. Washington, D.C.: National Academy Press.

International Centre for Diarrhoeal Disease Research, Bangladesh. (ICDDR,B). 1989. *Annual Report 1988*. Dhaka: ICDDR,B.

———. 1987. *Annual Report 1986*. Dhaka: ICDDR,B.

International Commission for the Study of Communication Problems. 1984. *Many Voices, One World: Communication and Society Today and Tomorrow* (the MacBride Report, abridged edition). United Kingdom: UNESCO.

International Development Research Centre. 1987. "Discussion Paper: Approaches to Strengthening Research Institutions." Ottawa: IDRC.

———. 1986. *Annual Report 1985-1986*. Ottawa: IDRC.

———. 1986.[a] *Multilateral Research Institutions in the Third World: A Directory of Multilateral Research and Research-Complementing Institutions Based in the Third World—1985*. Ottawa: IDRC.

———. 1986.[b] *With Our Own Hands—Research for Third*

World Development: Canada's Contribution Through the International Development Research Centre 1970-1985. Ottawa: IDRC.

International Fund for Agricultural Development. 1983. Nutritional Impact of Agricultural Projects, Rome.

International Health Policy Program (IHPP). 1989. "International Health Policy Program, An Introduction." Information Sheet, IHPP, S-6133. Washington, D.C.: IHPP.

International Monetary Fund. 1988. *International Financial Statistics Yearbook 1988.* Washington, D.C.: IMF.

International Service for National Agricultural Research. 1989. *1988 Annual Report.* The Hague: ISNAR.

Intersectoral Action for Health. 1987. *Report of the Intersectoral Action for Health Meeting on Health Objectives in Public Policy.* Cambridge, Mass., July 7-9, 1987. Geneva: WHO.

Japan International Cooperation Agency (JICA). 1987. *Annual Report 1987.* Tokyo: JICA.

W.K. Kellogg Foundation. 1987. *Annual Report 1986.* Battle Creek, Mich.: W.K. Kellogg Foundation.

Keyfitz, N. 1989. "The Growing Human Population." *Scientific American* 261 (September) 3:118-26.

————. 1982. *Population and Social Policy.* Cambridge, Mass: Abt Books.

Khon Kaen University, Faculty of Medicine. 1989. "Priority Problems in Curriculum Development." Technical Report. Khon Kaen, Thailand: Khon Kaen University.

Khorshid, M. 1988. "Cost-Effectiveness of Schistosomiasis Control Program in Egypt, with Special Emphasis on Community-based Health Education." In *Economics, Health and Tropical Diseases*, edited by A.N. Herrin and P.L. Rosenfield. Manila: University of the Philippines School of Economics.

Kidd, C.V., ed. 1980. *Biomedical Research in Latin America: Background Studies.* U.S. Department of Health, Education, and Welfare. Washington, D.C.: National Institutes of Health.

Kitron, U. 1989. "Integrated Disease Management of Tropical Infectious Diseases." In *International Cooperation for Health: Problems, Prospects, and Priorities*, edited by M.R. Reich and E. Marui. Dover Mass.: Auburn House.

Lasker, J. 1981. "Choosing Among Therapies: Illness Behaviour in the Ivory Coast." *Social Science and Medicine* 15(a):177-93.

Lechat, M.F. 1986. "Impact of Research and Technology on the Efficiency of Primary Health Care in Tropical Regions." Report prepared for the Commission of the European Communities Research Programme "Science and Technology for Development."

Lemma, A., and E. Valkonen, eds. 1987. *Towards National Capacity Building in Africa—University-Community Linkage for Child Survival and Development.* Finland: University of Helsinki—Lahti Research and Training Centre, and Florence, Italy: UNICEF International Child Development Centre.

Lewis, J.P. 1987. *External Funding of Development-Related Research: A Survey of Some Major Donors.* Ottawa: IDRC.

Lipton, M., and E. de Kadt. 1988. *Agricultural—Health Linkages.* Geneva: WHO.

Longhurst, R. 1984. *The Energy Trap: Work, Nutrition and Child Malnutrition in Northern Nigeria.* Cornell International Nutrition Monograph Series No. 13. Ithaca, N.Y.: Cornell University Press.

Lopez, A.D. 1989 (draft). "Causes of Death: An Assessment of Global and Regional Patterns of Mortality Around 1985." In *Evolving Health Sector Priorities in Developing Countries*, edited by D.J. Jamison and W.H. Mosley. Washington, D.C.: The World Bank Population, Health and Nutrition Department.

Lopez, A.D., and L.T. Ruzicka, eds. 1983. *Sex Differentials in Mortality: Trends, Determinants and Consequences.* Selection of the papers presented at the ANU/UN/WHO meeting held in Canberra, Australia, December 1-7, 1981. Miscellaneous Series No.4. Canberra: Department of Demography, Australian National University.

John D. and Catherine T. MacArthur Foundation. 1986. *Report on Activities 1986.* Chicago: John D. and Catherine T. MacArthur Foundation.

Madigan, F.C. 1988. "Key Issues Needing Attention with Regard to the Economics of Tropical Diseases." *Economics, Health and Tropical Diseases*, edited by A.N. Herrin and P.L. Rosenfield. Manila: University of the Philippines School of Economics.

Malikul, S. 1988. "The Need for Economic Research in Tropical Disease Control: the Control Program Perspective." In *Economics, Health and Tropical Diseases*, edited by A.N. Herrin and P.L. Rosenfield. Manila: University of the Philippines School of Economics.

Malo, S., and B. Gonzalez. 1988. "La convocatoria de 1988."

Ciencia y Desarrollo 14:101-7.

Malo, S. 1988. "La profesionalización de la investigación clínica." *Ciencia y Desarrollo* 14, 81:121-8.

Marmot, M., and T. Theorell. 1988. "Social Class and Cardiovascular Disease: The Contribution of Work." *International Journal of Health Services* 18, 4:659-74.

Martinez-Palomo, A. 1987. "Science for the Third World: An Inside View." *Perspectives in Biology and Medicine* 30, 4:546-57.

Martinez-Palomo, A., and J. Sepulveda. 1989. "Biomedical Research in Latin America: Old and New Challenges." *Annals of the New York Academy of Sciences.*

Mata, L., and L. Rosero. 1988. *National Health and Social Development in Costa Rica: A Case Study of Intersectoral Action.* Washington, D.C.: Pan American Health Organization.

Mauldin, W.P., and S. Segal. 1988. "Prevalence of Contraceptive Use: Trends and Issues." *Studies in Family Planning* 19, 6 (November-December).

Max, E. 1988. "Economics of Leprosy." *Economics, Health and Tropical Diseases.* Manila: University of the Philippines School of Economics.

May, P.R.A., B. Smedby, and L. Wetterberg, eds. 1986. "Perceptions of the Values and Benefits of Research: A Report by an International Study Group." *Acta Psychiatrica Scandinavica.* Supplementum No. 331, Vol. 74.

McCord, C., and H.P. Freeman. 1990. "Excess Mortality in Harlem." *New England Journal of Medicine* 322, 3:173-77.

McCracken, J., Conway, G. 1987. "Pesticide Hazards in the Third World: New Evidence from the Philippines." Gatekeeper Series No. SA1. London: International Institute for Environment and Development.

McKeigue, F.M., et al. 1988. "Diabetes, Hyperinsulinaemia, and Coronary Risk Factors in Bangladeshis in East London." *British Heart Journal* 60, 5:390-96.

Andrew W. Mellon Foundation. 1987. *Report of the Andrew W. Mellon Foundation 1987.* New York: Andrew W. Mellon Foundation.

Ministère des Relations Extérieures Coopération et Développement, France. 1986. *L'aide au Développement 1984-1985 Rapport D'Activité.* Paris: Ministère des Relations Extérieures Coopération et Développement.

Ministry of Health, Philippines. 1986. *Philippine Health Statistics, 1978-1984.* Philippines: Health Intelligence Service, MOH.

Ministry of Health, Zimbabwe. 1988. *Zimbabwe Epidemiological Bulletin* 18. Harare: Ministry of Health.

Ministry of Health and Family Welfare, Government of India. 1987. *Health Information of India.* New Delhi: Central Bureau of Health Intelligence, Government of India.

Ministry of Health and Welfare, Japan. 1987. *Health and Welfare Statistics in Japan.* Tokyo: Health and Welfare Statistics Association.

Ministry of Public Health, Thailand. *Public Health Statistics, 1982-1985.* Bangkok: Ministry of Public Health.

Ministry of Welfare, Health and Cultural Affairs. 1988. *Health Research Policy in the Netherlands.* Rijswijk: Department of Health Policy Development.

Mosley, W.H., D.T. Jamison, and D.A. Henderson. 1990 (forthcoming). "The Health Sector in Developing Countries: Problems for the 1990s and Beyond." *Annual Review of Public Health* 11.

Mosley, W.H., and C. Mauck. 1988 (April). "Technical Assistance: Professional Development and Career Structures in International Health." Paper presented at the Colloquium on International Health and Development in the 1990s. Baltimore, Md., The Johns Hopkins University School of Hygiene and Public Health.

Murray, C.J.L. 1990. "Mortality Among Black Men." Letter to the editor. *New England Journal of Medicine* 322, 3:205-06.

————. 1987. "A Critical Review of International Mortality Data." *Social Science and Medicine* 25, 7:773-81.

Murray, C.J.L., K. Styblo, and A. Rouillon. 1989. "Tuberculosis." *World Bank Health Sector Priorities Review.* Washington, D.C.: World Bank.

National Epidemiology Board of Thailand (NEBT). 1987. *Review of the Health Situation in Thailand: Priority Ranking of Diseases.* Thailand: NEBT.

Nichols, L., ed. 1982. "Science in Africa: Interviews with Thirty African Scientists." Washington, D.C.: Voice of America.

Norwegian Ministry of Development Cooperation (NORAD). 1987. *Norway's Assistance to Developing Countries in 1986.* Oslo: Development Assistance Committee, Memorandum of Norway.

Okita, S. 1988. "Rafael M. Salas Memorial Lecture 1988." New York: United Nations Population Fund.

Omran, A.R. 1971. "The Epidemiologic Transition: A Theory of the Epidemiology of Population Change." *Millbank Memorial Fund Quarterly* 49:509-38.

Organization for Economic Cooperation and Development. 1988. *Geographical Distribution of Financial Flows to Developing Countries—Disbursements, Commitments, Economic Indicators*. Paris, France: OECD.

————. 1985. *Measuring Health Care 1960-1983: Expenditure, Costs and Performance*. OECD Social Policy Studies No. 2. France: OECD.

————. 1981. *Support Funding for Biomedical Research in the OECD Area 1970-1980*. Paris: OECD.

Overseas Development Administration. 1987.[a] *Report on Research and Development 1986/87*. Central Office of Information, ODA.

————. 1987.[b] *British Aid Statistics 1982-1986: Statistics of UK Economic Aid to Developing Countries*. The Government Statistical Service.

————. 1984. *Second Report of Population Activities*. Central Office of Information, ODA.

————. (n.d.). *British Overseas Aid 1986*. Central Office of Information, ODA.

Overseas Development Council. 1989. "The Debate Over Intellectual Property: Whose Rights?" Congressional Staff Forum on International Development. Washington, D.C.: Overseas Development Council.

Pan American Health Organization (PAHO). 1987. *Research in Progress 1984, 1985*. Ref: RD 26/1. Washington, D.C.: PAHO.

Pardey, P.G., and J. Roseboom. 1989. *A Global Data Base on National Agricultural Research Systems*. ISNAR Agricultural Research Indicator Series. Cambridge: Cambridge University Press.

Perrin, L.H., P. Simitsek, and I. Srivastava. 1988. "Development of Malaria Vaccines." *Tropical and Geographical Medicine* 40, 3:S6-S21 (Supplement).

Pew Charitable Trusts. 1987. *Annual Report 1987*. Philadelphia: Pew Charitable Trusts.

————. 1986. *Annual Report 1986*. Philadelphia: Pew Charitable Trusts.

Pinstrup-Andersen, P. 1987. "Macroeconomic Adjustment and Human Nutrition" and "Macroeconomic Adjustment Policies and Human Nutrition: Available Evidence and Research Needs." Both in *Food and Nutrition Bulletin* 9 (March) 1.

Poikolainen, K. 1984. "Organization and Funding of Medical Research in 10 European Countries." *Scientometrics* 6, 5:327-58.

Popkin, B. 1978. "Nutrition and Labor Productivity." *Social Science and Medicine* 12C:117-25.

Preston, S.H. 1976. *Mortality Patterns in National Populations: With Special Reference to Recorded Causes of Death*. New York: Academic Press.

Ramalingaswami, V. 1989. "Importance of Vaccines in Child Survival," *Reviews of Infectious Diseases* 11 (Supplement 3)(May-June).

————. 1989.[a] "Asian Perspectives on the [AIDS] Epidemic." In *SIDA 2001, 22 et 23 Avril 1989*, edited by J.M. Dupuy, J.F. Lemaire, and L. Valette. Compte rendu de la réunion organisée aux Pensières a Veyrier-du-Lac ANNECY. ANNECY: Fondation Marcel Marieux, Fondation Universitaire des Sciences et Techniques du Vivant.

————. 1989.[b] "Vaccinology and the Goal of Health for All." In *Progress in Vaccinology*, edited by G.P. Talwar. New York: Springer-Verlag New York, Inc.

————. 1988. "Realistic Approaches—Looking Ahead Towards Comprehensive Rehabilitation." Sixteenth World Congress of Rehabilitation International, September 5-9, 1988. Tokyo: Rehabilitation International/Japanese Society for Rehabilitation of the Disabled/Japanese Association for Employment of the Disabled.

Repetto, R.C., ed. 1985. *The Global Possible: Resources, Development, and the New Century*. New Haven, Conn.: Yale University Press.

Rifkin, S.B. 1985. *Health Planning and Community Participation: Case Studies in Southeast Asia*. London: Croom Helm.

Rifkin, S.B., and G. Walt. 1986. "Why Health Improves: Defining the Issues Concerning 'Comprehensive Primary Health Care' and 'Selective Primary Health Care'." *Social Science and Medicine* 23, 6:559-66.

Robbins, A., and P. Freeman. 1988. "Obstacles to Developing

Vaccines for the Third World." *Scientific American* 256, 11:126-33.

Rockefeller Foundation. 1986. *1986 Annual Report*. New York: Rockefeller Foundation.

Rosenfield, P. 1986. "Linking Theory with Action: the Use of Social and Economic Research to Improve the Control of Tropical Parasitic Diseases." *Southeast Asian Journal of Tropical Medicine and Public Health* 17 (Sept.), 3:823-32.

Salam, A. 1989. *Notes on Science, Technology and Science Education in the Development of the South*. Prepared for the 5th Meeting of the South Commission, May 27-30, 1989, Maputo, Mozambique, and the meeting of the Heads of Government of the Non-Aligned Movement, September 4-7, 1989, Belgrade. Trieste: Third World Academy of Sciences.

Santos, A. 1988. "Economic Aspects Related to Schistosomiasis Transmission and Control." In *Economics, Health and Tropical Diseases*, edited by A.N. Herrin and P.L. Rosenfield. Manila: University of the Philippines School of Economics.

Sasakawa Memorial Health Foundation. 1989. *Leprosy Profiles with special attention to MDT Implementation*. Tokyo: Sasakawa Memorial Health Foundation.
Sasakawa Memorial Health Foundation. 1988. *Program Booklet*. Tokyo: Sasakawa Memorial Health Foundation.

Scrimshaw, N. 1989. "Infrastructure and Institution Building for Nutrition." Paper presented at a one-hour plenary session on August 25, 1989 at the 14th International Congress of Nutrition, Seoul, Korea.

———. 1984. "Functional Consequences of Iron Deficiency in Human Populations." *Journal of Nutritional Science and Vitaminology* 30:47-63.

SCRIP. *Pharmaceutical Company League Tables 1988*. 1988 (October). Surrey, U.K.: PJB Publications.

SEAMEO-TROPMED. 1989. *Fifth five-year plan of SEAMEO-TROPMED, July 1990-June 1995*. Bangkok: SEAMEO.

Sharma, G.K. 1988. "Use of Economics in Planning and Evaluating Disease Control Programmes." In *Economics, Health and Tropical Diseases*, edited by A.N. Herrin and P.L. Rosenfield. Manila: University of the Philippines School of Economics.
Shepard, D.S., and M.S. Thompson. 1979. "First Principles of Cost-effectiveness Analysis in Health." *Public Health Reports* 94:535-43.

Sitthi-amorn, C. 1989. "Assessment of Health Status: Whose

Viewpoints." Submitted to the *International Journal of Epidemiology*.

Smart, R. G., and G. F. Murray. 1985. "Narcotic Drug Abuse in 152 Countries: Social and Economic Conditions as Predictors." *The International Journal of the Addictions* 20, 5:737-49.

Smuckler, R.H., Berg, R.J., and D.F. Gordon. 1988. *New Challenges New Opportunities: U.S. Cooperation for International Growth and Development in the 1990s*. East Lansing, Mich.: Michigan State University.

Sommer, A., G. Hussaini, I. Tarwotjo, and D. Susanto. 1983. "Increased Mortality in Children with Mild Vitamin A Deficiency." *Lancet* 2:583-88.

Styblo, K. 1986. "Tuberculosis Control and Surveillance." In *Recent Advances in Respiratory Medicine*, edited by D.C. Flenley and T.L. Petty. New York: Churchill Livingstone.

Swedish Agency for Research Cooperation with Developing Countries (SAREC). 1989. *SAREC Annual Report 1987/88*. Stockholm: SAREC.

———. 1987. *SAREC's First Decade*. Stockhom: SAREC.

———. 1983. *National Research Councils in Developing Countries*. SAREC Seminar with Collaborating Agencies, Stockholm, Tammsuik, January 16-21, 1983. Stockholm: SAREC.

———. 1976. *SAREC's First Year Annual Report 1975–76*. Stockholm: SAREC.

Task Force for Child Survival. 1988. "Protecting the World's Children—An Agenda for the 1990s." Talloires, France (March 10- 12): The Task Force for Child Survival.

Third World Academy of Sciences. 1989. *Year Book of the Third World Academy of Sciences*. Italy: Third World Academy of Sciences.

Thrasher Research Fund. 1987. *Annual Report 1987*. Salt Lake City, Utah: Thrasher Research Fund.

Tjiptoherijanto. P., and R.M. Joesoef. 1988. "Epidemiological Model and Cost-effectiveness Analysis of Tuberculosis Treatment Programs in Indonesia." In *Economics, Health and Tropical Diseases*, edited by A.N. Herrin and P.L. Rosenfield. Manila: University of the Philippines School of Economics.

Tucker, S.K. 1989. "The Legacy of Debt: A Lost Decade of Development." *Policy Focus, No.3*. Background paper of the Overseas Development Council. Washington, D.C.: Overseas Development Council.

Tugwell, P., K.J. Bennett, D. Sackett, and B. Haynes. 1984. "Relative Risks, Benefits and Costs of Intervention." In *Tropical and Geographical Medicine*, edited by K. Warren and A. Mahmoud. New York: McGraw Hill.

Uchtenhagen, A. 1986. "Epidemiology and Trends in Narcotic and Psychotropic Drug Misuse and Related Problems." Conference of ministers of health on narcotic and psychotropic drug misuse. March 18-20, 1986. Geneva: WHO.

United Nations (UN). 1988. *World Population Prospects.* New York: UN.

———. 1986. *World Population Prospects: Estimates and Projections as Assessed in 1984.* Department of International Economic and Social Affairs, Population Studies, No. 98. New York: UN.

———. 1985. *Estimates and Projections of Urban, Rural and City Population, 1950-2025: the 1982 Assessment.* New York: Population Office, UN.

United Nations Administrative Committee on Coordination–Subcommittee on Nutrition. 1989. *Update on the Nutrition Situation: Recent Trends in Nutrition in 33 Countries.* Geneva: ACC/SCN at the World Health Organization.

———. 1987. *First Report on the World Nutrition Situation.* Geneva: ACC/SCN at WHO.

UNDP/World Bank/WHO Special Programme for Research and Training in Tropical Diseases (TDR). 1989. *Tropical Diseases—Progress in International Research, 1987-1988.* Ninth Programme Report. Geneva: WHO.

———. 1988. *New Approaches to Research Capability Strengthening.* Geneva: WHO.

———. 1987. *Tropical Disease Research: A Global Partnership*, edited by J. Maurice and A.M. Pearce. Geneva: WHO.

UNDP/UNFPA/World Bank/WHO Special Programme of Research, Development and Research Training in Human Reproduction (HRP). 1988. *Research in Human Reproduction: Biennial Report 1986-87.* Geneva: WHO.

———. 1985. *Fourteenth Annual Report, 1985.* Geneva: WHO.

UNESCO. 1986. *Human and Financial Resources for Research and Experimental Development in the Medical Sciences Division of Statistics on Science and Technology.* Office of Statistics, Paris: UNESCO.

UNICEF. 1989. *The State of the World's Children 1989.* New York: Oxford University Press.

United Nations Fund for Population Activities. 1988. *Guide to Sources of International Population Assistance—1988.* New York: UNFPA.

U.S. Agency for International Development (USAID). 1986 (December). *AID Policy Paper: Health Assistance.* Washington, D.C.: Bureau for Program and Policy Coordination, USAID.

———. 1986 (November). *User's Guide to the Office of Population USAID.* Office of Population, Bureau for Science and Technology, Washington, D.C.: USAID.

———. 1986. *Child Survival—A Second Report to Congress on the AID Program (Fiscal Year 1986).* Washington, D.C.: USAID.

United States Centers for Disease Control. 1986. "Premature Mortality in the United States: Public Health Issues in the Use of Years of Potential Life Lost." *Morbidity and Mortality Weekly Reports*, 35 (Supplement No. 25).

United States Department of Health and Human Services. 1985. *Health Status of Minorities and Low Income Groups.* DHHS Publication No. (HRSA) HRS-P-DV 85-1.

Vuthiponsge, P. 1989. "Institutional Capacity to Address Health Problems." In *International Cooperation for Health: Problems, Prospects, and Priorities*, edited by M.R. Reich and E. Marui. Dover, Mass.: Auburn House.

Walsh, J.A. 1988. *Establishing Health Priorities in the Developing World.* United Nations Development Programme, Division for Global and Interregional Programmes, New York: Adams Publishing Group.

Walsh, J.A., and K.S. Warren. 1986. *Strategies for Primary Health Care: Technologies Appropriate for the Control of Disease in the Developing World.* Chicago: University of Chicago Press.

———. 1979. "Selective Primary Health Care: An Interim Strategy for Disease Control in Developing Countries." *New England Journal of Medicine* 301:967-74.

Weisblat, A., and B. Kearl. 1989. "Building National Capacity in the Social Sciences: Insights from the Experience in Asia." Morrilton, Ark.: Winrock International Institute for Agricultural Development.

Wellcome Trust. 1987. *50 Years of the Wellcome Trust 1936–1986, Sixteenth Report 1984–1986.* London: Wellcome Trust.

Westcott, G. 1983. "Economics of Nutrition Planning." In *The Economics of Health in Developing Countries,* edited by K. Lee and A. Mills. Oxford: Oxford University Press.

Wheeler, J.C. 1987. *Development Co-operation: Efforts and Policies of the Members of the Development Assistance Committee.* Paris: OECD.

Wilson, R.G., J.H. Bryant, B.E. Echols, and A. Abrantes. 1988. *Management Information Systems and Microcomputers in Primary Health Care.* Report of an international workshop organized and sponsored by the Aga Khan Foundation, the Aga Khan University, and the National School of Public Health, Ministry of Health, Lisbon, Portugal. Conducted at the Gulbenkian Foundation Conference Centre, Lisbon, Portugal, November 1987. Aga Khan Foundation.

Winrock International. 1988. *Breaking the Cycle: Winrock International Annual Report 1987.* Morrilton, Ark.: Winrock International Institute for Agricultural Development.

Wolman, A. 1980. "Health and the Environment." *Bulletin of the Pan American Health Organization* 14, 1:6-14.

The World Bank. 1989. *World Development Report 1989.* New York: Oxford University Press.

———. 1988. *World Development Report 1988.* New York: Oxford University Press.

———. 1987. *The World Bank Atlas 1987.* Washington, D.C.: World Bank.

The World Commission on Environment and Development. 1987. *Our Common Future.* New York: Oxford University Press.

World Health Organization (WHO). 1988. *Alma-Ata Reaffirmed at Riga—A Statement of Renewed and Strengthened Commitment to Health for All by the Year 2000 and Beyond.* Report of the WHO meeting, Riga, U.S.S.R., March 22-25, 1988. From *Alma-Ata to the Year 2000: Reflections at the Midpoint.* Geneva: WHO.

———. 1988.[a] *Financial Report and Audited Financial Statements for the Financial Period 1 January 1986–31 December 1987, and Report of the External Auditor to the World Health Assembly.* Geneva: WHO.

———. 1988.[b] *Global Programme on AIDS—Progress Report Number 3.* Geneva: WHO.

———. 1988.[c] *Programme for the Control of Diarrhoeal Diseases.* Sixth Programme Report 1986-1987. Geneva: WHO.

———. 1988.[d] *Proposed Programme Budget for the Financial Period 1990–1991.* Geneva: WHO.

———. 1988.[e] *Proposed WHO Programme of Work in Health Economics, 1989–1991.* Unpublished manuscript. Geneva: WHO.

———. 1988.[f] *Strengthening Ministries of Health for Primary Health Care.* Report of a WHO Expert Committee. WHO Technical Report Series 766. Geneva: WHO.

———.1987. *Global Medium-Term Programme, Programme 3.3, Health Systems Research.* HSR/MTP/87.1. Geneva: WHO.

———. 1987.[a] *Global Review: An Evaluation of the Study of Health for All by the Year 2000.* Geneva: WHO.

———. 1987.[b] *Special Programme on AIDS—Strategies and Structure: Projected Needs.* Geneva: WHO.

———. 1986. *Proposed Programme Budget for the Financial Period 1988–1989.* Geneva: WHO.

———. 1982. *Tuberculosis Control.* Report of a Joint IUAT/WHO Study Group. Technical Report Series 671:1-26. Geneva: WHO.

———. 1978. *Primary Health Care.* Report of the International Conference on Primary Health Care, Alma-Ata, U.S.S.R., September 6-12, 1978. Geneva: WHO.

WHO Division of Strengthening of Health Services. 1988. *Health Economics: A Programme for Action.* Geneva: WHO.

———. 1988.[a] *Health Systems Research in Action.* Geneva: WHO.

———. 1988.[b] *Programme on Health Systems Research and Development.* Geneva: WHO.

WHO Expert Committee on Drug Dependence. 1989. *Twenty-sixth Report.* Technical Report Series 787. Geneva: WHO.

WHO Office of Research Promotion and Development. 1988. *WHO Research Activities: Biennium 1986-87.* Geneva: WHO.

World Resources Institute. 1987. *World Resources 1987: An Assessment of the Resource Base that Supports the Global Economy.* International Institute for Environment and Development, Washington, D.C.: World Resources Institute.

Yeon, H.C. 1989. "An Approach to Developing Primary Health Care in Korea." In *International Cooperation for Health: Problems, Prospects, and Priorities*, edited by M.R. Reich and E. Marui. Dover, Mass.: Auburn House.

Zurbrigg, S. 1984. "Rakku's Story: Structures of Ill-Health and Their Sources of Change." Madras: Madras Institute for Development Studies.

ABOUT THE COMMISSION

COMMISSION MEMBERS

John R. Evans *(Canada), Chair:* Chairman and chief executive officer of Allelix, Inc., a Canadian biotechnology firm; chairman of the Rockefeller Foundation; former director of the Department of Population, Health, and Nutrition of the World Bank; founding dean of the medical school at McMaster University (Canada); former president of the University of Toronto.

Gelia T. Castillo *(the Philippines), Deputy Chair:* Professor of rural sociology at the University of the Philippines, Los Baños; member of the board of governors of the International Development Research Centre (Canada), the WHO Scientific and Technical Advisory Committee for TDR (Special Programme for Research and Training in Tropical Diseases), and the Global Commission on AIDS.

Fazle Hasan Abed *(Bangladesh):* Founder and executive director of the Bangladesh Rural Advancement Committee (BRAC); winner of the 1980 Magsaysay Award for Community Leadership; chairman of the South Asia Partnership.

Sune D. Bergstrom *(Sweden):* Professor emeritus of biochemistry, Karolinska Institute in Stockholm; recipient of the 1982 Nobel Prize in Physiology or Medicine; former rector of the Karolinska Institute, former chair of the Nobel Foundation and the global Advisory Committee on Health Research of the World Health Organization.

Doris Howes Calloway *(United States):* Professor of nutrition and former provost of the professional schools and colleges at the University of California, Berkeley; member of the Institute of Medicine in the United States, the WHO's Expert Advisory Panel on Nutrition, and the Technical Advisory Committee (TAC) of the Consultative Group on International Agricultural Research (CGIAR).

Essmat S. Ezzat *(Egypt):* Co-founder of the medical school, dean of the faculty of medicine, and professor of internal medicine, Suez Canal University, Ismailia; member of the Federation of Medical Education and the International Clinical Epidemiology Network (INCLEN).

Demissie Habte *(Ethiopia):* Professor of pediatrics and child health and former dean of the medical school, Addis Ababa University; director of the International Centre for Diarrheal Disease Research, Bangladesh.

Walter J. Kamba *(Zimbabwe):* Vice chancellor and professor of law, University of Zimbabwe; former dean of the faculty of law, University of Dundee (Scotland); member of the board of governors and the executive committee of the International Development Research Centre (Canada).

Adetokunbo O. Lucas *(Nigeria):* Chair of the Carnegie Corporation's Strengthening Human Resources in Developing Countries Program; former professor of preventive and social medicine, University of Ibadan (Nigeria); former director of the UNDP/World Bank/WHO Special Programme for Research and Training in Tropical Diseases (TDR).

Adolfo Martinez-Palomo *(Mexico):* Professor of cell biology at the National Polytechnical Institute, Mexico City; winner of the 1988 Third World Academy of Sciences award in biology; member of the executive council of the Latin American Academy of Sciences, the board of governors of the National University of Mexico, and the Third World Academy of Sciences.

Saburo Okita *(Japan):* Former foreign minister of Japan; member of the Pearson Commission (1968-69), and the Brundtland Commission (1985-88); chairman, advisory committee on international development cooperation to the prime minister of Japan; chancellor, International University of Japan; advisor to the Environment Agency; chairman, World Institute for Development Economics Research of the United Nations University; and chairman, Japan UNICEF Committee.

V. Ramalingaswami *(India):* Special advisor to the executive director of UNICEF; former director of the All India Institute of Medical Sciences, former director-general of the Indian Council for Medical Research; former chair, global Advisory Committee on Health Research of the World Health Organization; adjunct professor of international health policy at the Harvard School of Public Health.

SPONSORS OF
THE COMMISSION

Academia de la Investigacion Cientifica, Mexico
The Carnegie Corporation of New York, United States
The Edna McConnell Clark Foundation, United States
The Ford Foundation, United States
Foundation for Total Health Promotion, Japan
Gesellschaft für Technische Zusammenarbeit, Federal Republic of Germany
The International Development Research Centre, Canada
The Nobel Assembly, Sweden
The Oak Foundation, United Kingdom
The Overseas Development Administration, United Kingdom
The Pew Charitable Trusts, United States
The Rockefeller Foundation, United States
Swedish Agency for Research Cooperation with Developing Countries
Swiss Development Cooperation and Humanitarian Aid
The United Nations Development Programme
The World Bank

The Commission has, in addition, received support from
the following for workshops and meetings:

Advisory Board in Epidemiology, Mexico
Bangladesh Rural Advancement Committee
Directorate-General of Epidemiology, Mexico
Harvard University, United States
The Hinduja Foundation, United States
Government of Japan, Ministry of Foreign Affairs
Government of the State of Mexico, Ministry of Health
Government of the State of Mexico, Office of the Governor
Government of Zimbabwe, Ministry of Health
International Congress for Tropical Medicine and Malaria
Japan International Cooperation Agency
Organization of American States
Oswaldo Cruz Institute, Brazil
Pan American Health Organization, Regional Office for the Americas
        of the World Health Organization
Royal Tropical Institute, the Netherlands
Southern African Development Coordination Conference
South Asian Association for Regional Cooperation
The United Nations Children's Fund
University of Zimbabwe

COMMISSION SECRETARIAT

The main office of the Commission secretariat is:

Commission on Health Research for Development
22 Plympton Street
Cambridge, MA 02138, United States

Telephone: (617) 495-8498
Fax: (617) 495-5418
Telex: 415313

Cambridge, Massachusetts, U.S.A.
Lincoln C. Chen *(United States), Study Director:* Taro Takemi Professor of International Health at the Harvard School of Public Health and director of the Harvard Center for Population Studies.
David E. Bell *(United States), Senior Consultant:* Clarence Gamble Professor of Population Sciences and International Health, emeritus, at the Harvard School of Public Health.

London, United Kingdom
Richard G. Feachem *(United Kingdom), Senior Consultant:* Dean of the London School of Hygiene and Tropical Medicine; former Principal Public Health Specialist, World Bank.
David J. Bradley, *(United Kingdom), Senior Consultant:* Director, Ross Institute, London School of Hygiene and Tropical Medicine.

Tokyo, Japan
Shigekoto Kaihara *(Japan), Senior Consultant:* Chairman, Division of International Health, Faculty of Medicine, Tokyo University.
Eiji Marui, *(Japan), Consultant:* Assistant Professor, Division of International Health, Faculty of Medicine, Tokyo University.

STAFF OF THE SECRETARIAT

For varying periods of time, the following have worked for the secretariat:

Sunil Chacko *(India), Assistant Director*
Erik De Jonghe *(Belgium), Commission survey*
Gary Gleason *(United States), Communication*
Jill Kneerim *(United States), Editor*
Catherine Michaud *(Switzerland), Country studies*
Christopher J.L. Murray *(New Zealand), Staff economist, Commission survey*
Evelyn Rosenthal *(United States), Copyeditor*
Stephen Tollman *(United Kingdom), Essential national health research*
Alberto Torres *(Spain), Research, drafting*
Elissa Weitzman *(United States), Research, drafting*
Sarah Zaidi *(Pakistan), Commission survey*

Research Staff
Asif Aslam *(Pakistan)*
Eunice Ndajigimana *(Uganda)*
Karen Peterson *(United States)*
Xinjian Qiao *(China)*
Alvaro Tinajero *(Ecuador)*
Javier Vidal *(Spain)*

Administrative Staff
Linda Bennett
Emily Haslett
Janet Kresge
Michelle MacKenzie
Sally Martin
Kelly Ward
Ron Ward

DESIGN AND PRODUCTION OF THIS BOOK WERE DONE BY QBC SYSTEMS, RIVER EDGE, NEW JERSEY

COMMISSION ACTIVITIES

COMMISSION MEETINGS

1) Bad Soden, Federal Republic of Germany—November 4-7, 1987.
2) Harare, Zimbabwe—January 26-29, 1988.
3) Cambridge, Massachusetts, United States—May 21-23, 1988.
4) Mexico City, Mexico—September 2-4, 1988.
5) New Delhi, India—January 7-9, 1989.
6) Tokyo, Japan—June 19-21, 1989.
7) Paris, France—November 28-29, 1989.
8) Stockholm, Sweden—February 21-23, 1990.

COLLABORATIVE WORKSHOPS

1) Ottawa, Canada: International Development Research Centre (IDRC), March 20-21, 1989.
2) Dhaka, Bangladesh: Bangladesh Rural Advancement Committee in cooperation with SAARC, June 25-27, 1989.
3) Harare, Zimbabwe: University of Zimbabwe in cooperation with SADCC, August 17-19, 1989.
4) Hamilton, Canada: McMaster University Medical School, September 7, 1989.
5) Rio de Janeiro, Brazil: Oswaldo Cruz Foundation in cooperation with the Pan American Health Organization, October 10-12, 1989.
6) Amsterdam, the Netherlands: Royal Tropical Institute in cooperation with European colleagues, November 30-December 1, 1989.
7) Cairo, Egypt: Suez Canal University Medical School in cooperation with the National Academy of Sciences, Egypt, December 2-4, 1989.
8) Puebla, Mexico: Ministry of Health, Government of Mexico in cooperation with the Advisory Board in Epidemiology, Mexico, the Pan American Health Association, and the Organization of American States, January 18-19, 1990.

SECRETARIAT WORKSHOPS

1) Approaches to Capacity Building—December 9, 1987.
2) Capacity Strengthening Strategies—January 5, 1988.
3) Health Policy Research—April 19, 1988.
4) Health and Mortality Data—April 28, 1988.
5) Health Economics (London)—May 5, 1988.
6) Epidemiology and Field Research—August 15, 1988.
7) Mental Health and Health Behavior—November 28, 1988.

8) Micronutrient Deficiencies—December 8-9, 1988.
9) Essential National Research—February 27-28, 1989.
10) Tuberculosis Research—September 18, 1989.
11) Meetings of the Okita Committee (Tokyo)—May 2, 1988; June 20, 1988; August 22, 1988; December 6, 1988; April 21, 1989; June 19, 1989; September 15, 1989; December 22, 1989; January 11, 1990.

CONSULTATIVE ACTIVITIES

Developing-country consultations Extensive consultations have been conducted with over 1,000 scientists, governmental leaders, social activists, and professionals around the world. Very strong participation was obtained from developing-country leaders through in-country workshops and extensive travel by commissioners and staff. During Commission meetings and workshops, open forums have been conducted inviting a broad range of comments and suggestions from interested parties.

International agencies Regular communications and discussions have been pursued with key international agencies, including the senior leadership of WHO, UNICEF, UNDP, UNESCO, UNFPA, the World Bank, and regional associations such as the Commonwealth Secretariat, SAARC, and SADCC.

Professional community Commissioners and staff have met with numerous professional associations, such as the Third World Academy of Sciences, the African Academy of Sciences, the International Conference for Tropical Medicine and Malaria, the International Union Against Tuberculosis, the International Epidemiological Association, the National Council for International Health (United States) and the Board on International Health, Institute of Medicine (United States).

Donor discussions The Commission is sponsored by 16 agencies. In 1988, the Commission conducted separate briefing sessions for North American and European donors and in 1989 donor discussions were pursued in Japan.

ACKNOWLEDGMENTS

In two years' work, the Commission has consulted widely with people around the world. We list below those who have contributed to the formation of our vision. We regret that we have not been able to record the name of every person who has been of help to the Commission and apologize for any omissions or errors in this list.

Amir Abbas, Egypt
Wajaa Abdalla, Egypt
Hussein Abd el Aziz, Egypt
M. Abdelmoumene, Intl.
Ibraheem Helmy Abdurrahman, Egypt
Ragaa Abdurrassul, Egypt
Brian Abel-Smith, U.K.
Ela Abraham, India
Taha Abushoosha, Egypt
Oscar Mateo de Acosta, Cuba
Fathy Afia, Egypt
Kamaluddin Ahmed, Bangladesh
Salehuddin Ahmed, Bangladesh
Akwasi Aidoo, Tanzania
Iain Aitken, U.K.
Shawky el Akabawy, Egypt
Halida Akhtar, Bangladesh
John Akin, U.S.A.
Elizabeth Alger, U.S.A.
Mohammed Hag Ali, Sudan
Alberto Alzate, Colombia
N. H. Antia, India
Jose Aponte, U.S.A.
Hugo Aréchiga, Mexico
Mario Argandona-Yanez, Bolivia
Michael Arkin, Canada
Edward Arnold, U.S.A.
Guillermo Arroyave, Guatemala

Deanna Ashley, Jamaica
William Asenso, Ghana
E. Assey, Tanzania
Antoine Augustin, Haiti
James Austin, U.S.A.
Philippe Authier, Belgium
Fouad Badr, Egypt
Ibraheem Badran, Egypt
Charles Bailey, U.S.A.
Jane Baltazar, Philippines
G. Bango, Zimbabwe
Z. Bankowski, Intl.
Pranab Bardhan, India
Carol Barker, U.K.
Geoff Barnard, U.K.
B. F. Baron, U.S.A.
Kenneth Bart, U.S.A.
Jose Barzelatto, Chile
Samir Basta, Intl.
V. Bavanandan, Malaysia
LeAnn Beebe, U.S.A.
Syeda Feroza Begum, Bangladesh
Kert Beiersdorfer, F.R.G.
Peter Bell, U.S.A.
Bo Bengtsson, Sweden
Alfredo Bengzon, Philippines
Michael Bennish, U.S.A.
Arturo Beltran, Mexico

Alan Berg, U.S.A.
Susan Berger, U.S.A.
Lucien Bernard, France
Munevver Bertan, Turkey
Guido Bertolaso, Italy
Andrew Beyer, U.S.A.
Natth Bhamarapravati, Thailand
Ela Bhatt, India
Julia Chang Block, U.S.A.
Jose-Luis Bobadilla, Mexico
Pierre Bois, Canada
Binger Borregaard, Denmark
Carmen Borosso, Brazil
Abdel Wahid Bosseila, Egypt
Nyle Brady, U.S.A.
John Briscoe, Intl.
Arthur Brown, Jamaica
George Brown, U.S.A.
Graham Brown, Australia
Jean Brouste, France
Hector Brust, Mexico
Anne Bruzelius, Sweden
Al Buck, U.S.A.
Stewart Burden, U.S.A.
B. Meredith Burke, U.S.A.
William Butler, U.S.A.
Mayra Buvinic, U.S.A.

Jorge Cabral, Mozambique
Jin-Wen Cai, People's Republic of China
John Caldwell, Australia
Pat Caldwell, Australia
Juan Calva, Mexico
Erney Camargo, Brazil
Fernando Cano, Mexico
Andre Capron, France
R. E. Cardinal, Canada
C. A. Carlaw, Zimbabwe
Patrizia Carlevaro, U.S.A.
Guy Carrin, Belgium
Richard Cash, U.S.A.
Margaret Catley-Carlson, Canada
Jackie Cattani, Intl.
Carlos Chagas, Brazil
N. T. Chaibva, Zimbabwe
S. K. Chandiwana, Zimbabwe
Mirai Chatterji, India
Federico Chávez, Mexico
Manuel Ruiz de Chavez, Mexico

Evgeny Chazov, U.S.S.R.
C. J. Chetsanga, Zimbabwe
N. T. Chideya, Zimbabwe
R. M. Chimba, Zambia
T. M. Chimbadzwa, Zimbabwe
P. C. Chimimba, Malawi
Changen Choprapawon, Thailand
A. Mushtaq R. Chowdhury, Bangladesh
Kamla Chowdhry, India
S. G. M. Chowdhury, Bangladesh
T. A. Chowdhury, Bangladesh
Zafrullah Chowdhury, Bangladesh
Julie Cliff, Mozambique
Wilbur Colburn, U.S.A.
Bill Connelly, U.S.A.
Joseph A. Cook, U.S.A.
Diana Cooper-Weil, U.S.A.
Manuel Corachan, Spain
Immita Cornaz, Switzerland
Deborah Cotton, U.S.A.
Banoo Coyaji, India
Andrew Creese, Intl.
George Cumper, U.K.

Doug Daniels, Canada
Henry Danielson, Sweden
Monica Das Gupta, India
John David, U.S.A.
James Dawson, U.S.A.
James Deane, U.K.
Mark De Bruycker, Belgium
Anwar el Deeb, Egypt
Aubine Degremont, Switzerland
Anil Deolalikar, India
Helmut Determann, F.R.G.
W. J. De Voogt, the Netherlands
M. Dickens, U.K.
Letticia Diescho, South Africa
H. J. Diesfield, F.R.G.
William Draper, Intl.
General Durand, France
Ramesh Durvasula, India
D. Duwel, F.R.G.

Tony Earls, U.S.A.
Rosemary Eder-Debye, F.R.G.
Joanne Edgar, U.S.A.
Roger Eeckels, Belgium
Thomas Egwang, Uganda

Leon Eisenberg, U.S.A.
Same Ekobo, Cameroon
Andrea Eschen, U.S.A.
G. M. van Etten, the Netherlands
L. Eyckmans, Belgium

G. Samdani Fakir, Bangladesh
Olfat Farag, Egypt
Rifky Faris, Egypt
M. F. Fathalla, Intl.
Anibal Faundes, Brazil
David Feeny, Canada
Isabel Fezer, F.R.G.
Harvey Fineberg, U.S.A.
Sally Findley, U.S.A.
C. Fischer, F.R.G.
Jean-Marc Fleury, Canada
Amador Flores, Mexico
Rafael Flores, Guatemala
William Foege, U.S.A.
Ingrid Foik, F.R.G.
Thomas Fox, U.S.A.
Lennart Freij, Sweden
Julio Frenk, Mexico
Dominique Frommel, Norway
Juan Ramon de la Fuente, Mexico
K. Fukai, Japan
Naoki Furuta, Japan

Barry Gaberman, U.S.A.
Rajiv Gandhi, India
B. C. Garg, India
Ann Gardner, U.S.A.
Michel Garenne, France
Peter Geithner, U.S.A.
Hellen Gelband, U.S.A.
Marc Gentillini, France
John Gerhart, U.S.A.
Haider Ghaleb, Egypt
Duff Gillespie, U.S.A.
Jeff Gimbel, U.S.A.
Tore Godal, Intl.
Peter Goldmark, U.S.A.
C. Gopalan, India
James P. Grant, Intl.
Marcus Grant, Intl.
L. Grauls, Belgium
Adrianne Grunberg, U.S.A.
Rodrigo Guerrero, Colombia

Samir Guirguis, Egypt
Gonzalo Gutiérrez, Mexico
Davidson Gwatkin, U.S.A.

Mustafa Habib, Egypt
Jean-Pierre Habicht, U.S.A.
G. Gordon Hadley, U.S.A.
Saleh el Hak, Egypt
Scott Halstead, U.S.A.
Salah Hamady, Egypt
Laiila el Hamamsy, Egypt
David Hamburg, Intl.
Ann Hamilton, U.S.A.
Hammam Hammam, Egypt
Mustafa Hammouda, Egypt
Tertit von Hanno Aasland, Norway
A. C. Harid, Zimbabwe
Oscar Harkavy, U.S.A.
Kelsey Harrison, Nigeria
Roger Harrison, U.K.
Frank Hartvelt, Intl.
Toshihiko Hasegawa, Japan
Ivan Head, Canada
Nabila Hedayet, Egypt
Donald Henderson, U.S.A.
Rafe Henderson, Intl.
Caroline Hernández, Canada
Mauricio Hernandez, Mexico
F. W. G. Hill, Zimbabwe
David Hilton, U.K.
James Himes, U.S.A.
H. B. Himonga, Zambia
Dan Holzner, U.S.A.
Thavitong Hongvivatana, Thailand
David Hopper, Canada
Shiro Horiuchi, Japan
Mary Horner, U.S.A.
Manowar Hossain, Bangladesh
Lucien Houllemare, France
O. E. M. Hove, Zimbabwe
Robert Hughes, U.S.A.
Valerie Hull, Australia
David Hunter, Australia
Munimul Huq, Bangladesh
S. Huq, Bangladesh
A. M. Z. Hussain, Bangladesh
M. Hussain, Bangladesh

Barbara Ibraheem, Egypt

Yutaka Iimura, Japan
Shozo Iizawa, Japan
Hiroyuki Ishi, Japan
N. Ishikawa, Japan
Nurul Islam, Bangladesh
Wahidul Islam, Bangladesh
Edda Ivan-Smith, U.K.

Ibrahim Jabr, Intl.
Brunet Jailly, Mali
Devaki Jain, India
M. A. Jalil, Bangladesh
John James, U.K.
Dean Jamison, U.S.A.
José Jessurum, Mexico
Cai Jin-wen, China
T. Jacob John, India
Pamela Johnson, U.S.A.
Lloyd Johnston, U.S.A
Richard Jolly, Intl.

Sandra Kabir, Bangladesh
Somkid Kaewsonthi, Thailand
K. Kalumba, Zambia
Arjumand Kamal, Pakistan
Medhat Kamal, Egypt
M. Kamaluddin, Bangladesh
Aissata Kane, Mauritania
Y. Kaneko, Japan
Phyllis Kanki, U.S.A.
L. Kaptué, Cameroon
Frank Karel, U.S.A.
Dan Kaseje, Kenya
C. A. Kauser, Bangladesh
Y. Kawaguchi, Intl.
Tsuneaki Kawamura, Japan
A. B. M. Najmul Kawnine, Bangladesh
Derege Kebede, Ethiopia
Barbara Kelly, U.K.
Anthony Kennedy, U.S.A.
Barbara Kehrer, U.S.A.
Susi Kessler, Intl.
Mohd. Khalilullah, Bangladesh
Nagwa Khallaf, Egypt
A. K. Azad Khan, Bangladesh
Karim Aga Khan, France
M. R. Khan, Bangladesh
Aly Khater, Egypt
Tymoor Khattab, Egypt

Ishak el Khawashgy, Egypt
Ahmed Khorsheid, Egypt
P. Khulumani, Botswana
Kenzo Kiikuni, Japan
W. L. Kilama, Tanzania
Charles Kinbote, Zembla
S. N. Kinoti, Kenya
Kabiru Kinyanjui, Kenya
Tadao Kishi, Japan
Arthur Kleinman, U.S.A.
Karl-Eric Knuttson, Intl.
Arata Kochi, Japan
Amadou Koita, Mali
Riitta-Liisa Kolehmainen-Aitken, Finland
Takefumi Kondo, Japan
Rolf Korte, F.R.G.
Jan Kostrzewski, Poland
Wilhelm Krull, F.R.G.
Jesus Kumate, Mexico

Paul Ladouceur, Intl.
Sandra Lane, U.S.A.
Richard Laing, Zimbabwe
Mary Ann Lansang, Philippines
John Lawrence, U.S.A.
Ernst Lauridsen, Denmark
Kenneth Lee, U.K.
Aklilu Lemma, Intl.
Joanne Leslie, U.S.A.
Richard Levins, U.S.A.
Angel Lezana, Mexico
Gustaaf W. von Liebenstein, the Netherlands
Bernhard Liese, Intl.
Phyllis Lightfoot, U.S.A.
Khor Geok Lin, Malaysia
Alf Lindberg, Sweden
Jorge Litvak, U.S.A.
Borje Ljunggren, Sweden
Rene Loewenson, Zimbabwe
Alan Lopez, Intl.
Malaquias López, Mexico
Andrea Loyola, Brazil

Kurt-Jurgen Maab, F.R.G.
Rufino Macagba, U.S.A.
P. Mackenbach, the Netherlands
Salah Madkour, Egypt
Ignacio Madrazo, Mexico
Dilip Mahalanabis, India

Halfdan Mahler, Denmark
M. P. Makhubu, Swaziland
Daniel Makuto, Zimbabwe
G. M. Malahleha, Lesotho
M. A. Malek, Bangladesh
G. M. Mandishona, Zimbabwe
F. Manji, Kenya
B. Mansourian, Intl.
B. Manyame, Zimbabwe
Jaime Martuscelli, Mexico
Ghassan Master, Lebanon
V. I. Mathan, India
J. K. G. Mati, Kenya
Yves Matillon, France
Hitoshi Matsuoka, Japan
Kouichiro Matsuura, Japan
Emmanuel Max, India
Federico Mayor, Intl.
Rika Mazaki, Japan
L. Mbengeranwa, Zimbabwe
Robert McDonoygh, U.S.A.
William McDougal, U.S.A.
Don McKibben, Canada
Anthony Measham, Intl.
Martha Medina, Nicaragua
Anne Melgaard, Denmark
J.B. Mendis, Intl.
Alfred Merkle, F.R.G.
Michael Merson, Intl.
Fisseha Meskal, Ethiopia
D. G. Metcalfe, U.K.
Simon Metcalfe, Zimbabwe
Robert Meyers, U.S.A.
Marvelous Mhloyi, Zimbabwe
Anne Mills, U.K.
Jean-Francois Minder, France
Howard Miners, U.S.A.
Eduardo Missoni, Italy
Dade Moeller, U.S.A.
Edgar Mohs, Costa Rica
S. Mombeshora, Zimbabwe
Humberto Montiel, Nicaragua
Dolores Moran, Ireland
Carlos Morel, Brazil
Carlos Moreno, Mexico
Iwao Moriyama, U.S.A.
Richard Morrow, U.S.A.
Henry Mosley, U.S.A.
Jean Mouchet, France

John Mramba, Kenya
L. A. H. Msukwa, Malawi
N. O. Mugwagwa, Zimbabwe
Eustace Muhondwa, Tanzania
Daleep Mukarji, India
Alok Mukhopadhyay, India
K. Mukunyandela, Zambia
Alexander Muller, the Netherlands
Toshio Murakoshi, Japan
M. W. Murphree, Zimbabwe
Colleen Murphy, U.S.A.
Nirmala Murthy, India
R. Srinivasa Murthy, India
Stanley Music, U.S.A.
Michio Mutaguchi, Japan
J. Mutambirwa, Zimbabwe
Germano Mwabu, Kenya
Jonathan Myers, South Africa

David Nabarro, U.K.
M. A. Najeeb, Pakistan
Hiroshi Nakajima, Intl.
Eiichi Nakamura, Japan
Heba Nassar, Egypt
Shajika Nasser, Egypt
Lalit Nath, India
D. Ncube, Zimbabwe
M. Ncube, Zimbabwe
Courtney Nelson, U.S.A.
Victor Neufeld, Canada
Kenneth Newell, U.K.
Jacob Ngu, Cameroon
N. Nhlabatsi, Swaziland
A. M. Nhonoli, Tanzania
Ole Frank Nielson, Denmark
K. Nishioka, Japan
Yoshiyuki Nishizawa, Japan
Rukarangira Wa Nkere, Zaire
J. C. Nkomo, Zimbabwe
F. K. Nkrumah, Ghana
Zohair Nooman, Egypt
David Nostbakken, Canada
Yvo Nuyens, Intl.
M. Nxumalo, Swaziland
B.B. Nyathi, Zimbabwe

Michio Obata, Japan
Joe Odhiambo, Kenya
Thomas Odhiambo, Kenya

Ingrid Ofstad, Norway
Orla O'Hanrahan, Ireland
Teresa O'Hara, Ireland
Helen Ohlin, Sweden
Chinyelu Okafor, Nigeria
Onesmo Ole-Moiyoi, Kenya
Kazuyuki Omae, Japan
A. H. S. Omer, Sudan
L. O. Omondi, Botswana
Takao Onishi, Japan
Jose Oquendo, U.S.A.
Manuel Ortega, Mexico
Tom Ortiz, U.S.A.
Maged Osman, Egypt
Nils Ostrom, Sweden
Ait Ouyahia, Algeria
C. O. Oyejide, Nigeria

Saroj Pachauri, India
B. Pannenborg, the Netherlands
Gaspar Garcia de Paredes, Panama
Edward Pariaga, U.S.A.
Alan Parker, U.K.
Mukesh Patel, India
Ashok Patil, India
G. Paul-Mechel, F.R.G.
Bernard Philipon, France
Margaret Phillips, U.K.
Marina Pearce, U.K.
Nate Pierce, Intl.
Martha Piña, Mexico
Per Pinstrup-Andersen, U.S.A.
Jacqueline Pitanguy, Brazil
Sam Pitroda, India
Christina Possas, Brazil
Joseph Potter, U.S.A.
Z. Powlowski, Poland
Dennis Prager, U.S.A.
Willard de Pree, U.S.A.
Kenneth Prewitt, U.S.A.
K. Pulst, F.R.G.

M. S. Qasem, Bangladesh
Mml. Quesada, Philippines
Asma Fozia Qureshi, Pakistan

G. S. Rahman, Bangladesh
Kazi Masihur Rahman, Bangladesh
M. Omar Rahman, Bangladesh
M. B. Rahman, Bangladesh

T. Rahman, Bangladesh
K. Rajagopalan, India
V. K. Ramachandran, India
T. Ramatlapeng, Lesotho
Jairam Ramesh, India
Rafael Ramos, Mexico
Mamphela Ramphele, South Africa
O. Ransome-Kuti, Nigeria
Amany Refaat, Egypt
Michael Reich, U.S.A.
Lance M. Renault, U.S.A.
Susan Rifkin, U.S.A.
Rebecca Rimel, U.S.A.
Federico Ritcher, Guatemala
Fareg Rizk, Egypt
Juan Rivera, Guatemala
Luis Rivera, U.S.A.
Zia Rizvi, Pakistan
Yves Robin, France
Patricia Rosenfield, U.S.A.
J. Ross, U.S.A.
E. Rost, F.R.G.
Alessandro Rossi-Espagnet, Italy
Timothy Rothermel, Intl.
Annik Rouillon, France
Avery Russell, U.S.A.
William Rust, U.S.A.

Muhammad Saber, Egypt
M. Sachikonye, Zimbabwe
Samira Sadik, Egypt
Fred Sai, Intl.
Abdus Salam, Intl.
Ebrahim Samba, Intl.
Jacques Sant'Ana Calazans, France
Carlos Santos, Mexico
Norman Sartorius, Intl.
Plearnpit Satsanguan, Thailand
PleaHamdy el Sayed, Egypt
Allan Schapira, Denmark
Nevin Scrimshaw, U.S.A.
Sheldon Segal, U.S.A.
Amartya Sen, India
Jaime Sepulveda, Mexico
W. Frederick Shaw, U.S.A.
James Shelton, U.S.A.
Donald Shepard, U.S.A.
Ahmed Fouad el Sherbeini, Egypt
Mitsuo Shikano, Japan
Tadao Shimao, Japan

M. Shiva, Zimbabwe
Nadya Shmavonian, U.S.A.
A. T. Siddiqui, Bangladesh
G. G. Sikipa, Zimbabwe
D. R. Silimperi, U.S.A.
Alberto Carvalho da Silva, Brazil
Jonathan Simon, U.S.A.
Stephen Simon, Canada
Manmohan Singh, India
Chitr Sitthi-amorn, Thailand
M. Slaoui, Switzerland
Lewis Slotin, Canada
Karl Smith, Canada
R. H. M. Smulders, the Netherlands
Guillermo Soberon, Mexico
K. Soels, the Netherlands
Orville Solon, Philippines
Edith Sonntag, U.S.A.
Sumarmo Soedarmo, Indonesia
Sergio Spinaci, Italy
John Stanbury, U.S.A.
Goran Sterky, Sweden
Jill Steward, U.K.
Sir Kenneth Stewart, Jamaica
Don Stilwell, U.S.A.
Peter Streefland, the Netherlands
H. Streibel, Switzerland
P. A. Stroberg, the Netherlands
Karel Styblo, Czechoslovakia
Jonathan Sugar, U.S.A.
G. Szczerban, Intl.

Nebiat Tafari, Ethiopia
Kazuo Takahashi, Japan
Hiroshi Takeda, Japan
Keizo Takemi, Japan
M. K. Talukder, Bangladesh
Marcel Tanner, Switzerland
Roberto Tapia, Mexico
Randi Tasserud, Norway
Munir Tawal, Egypt
Floyd Taylor, U.S.A.
Paul Taylor, Zimbabwe
Wilfried P. Thalwitz, Intl.
Adolf Tham, Sweden
Carl Tham, Sweden
Vinod Thomas, India
Irene Tinker, U.S.A.
Alison Tipping, U.K.
H. Torloni, Brazil
T. S. Tswana, Zimbabwe
Peter Tugwell, Canada

J. Ellis Turner, U.S.A.

Itoka J. Udeinya, Nigeria
Naruo Uehara, Japan
Mukund Uplekar, India

José Valdespino, Mexico
Giuseppe Valentini, Italy
John Vanderveen, U.S.A.
Ann Van Dusen, U.S.A.
Fernando Cano Valle, Mexico
Marlon Verasamy, U.S.A.
C. Varkevisser, the Netherlands
Rafael Velasco, Mexico
Aurora Velazquez, Nicaragua
P. B. Vengesa, Zimbabwe
R. Venkataraman, India
Mechai Viravaidya, Thailand
Tarzie Vittachie, Sri Lanka
My Vu, Vietnam

Catriona Waddington, U.K.
Takashi Wagatsuma, Japan
Youssef Waheeb, Egypt
F. Waldeck, F.R.G.
Ron Waldman, U.S.A.
M. Waliullah, Bangladesh
Dave Walker, U.S.A.
Julia Walsh, U.S.A.
B. Wangman, Nigeria
Janet Wardlaw, Canada
Kenneth Warren, U.S.A.
Peter Way, U.S.A.
Karl Western, U.S.A.
Mark Wheeler, U.K.
Roy Widdus, Intl.
Walter Willet, U.S.A.
Van Williams, U.S.A.
Richard Wilson, Canada
Jay Winsten, U.S.A.
Joseph Wray, U.S.A.
Susan Wray, Jamaica
John Wyon, U.K.

Xu Xiping, China

Kensuke Yanagiya, Japan

Barbara de Zalduondo, U.S.A.
Pacita Zara, Philippines
George Zeidenstein, U.S.A.
Huda Zurayk, Egypt

INDEX